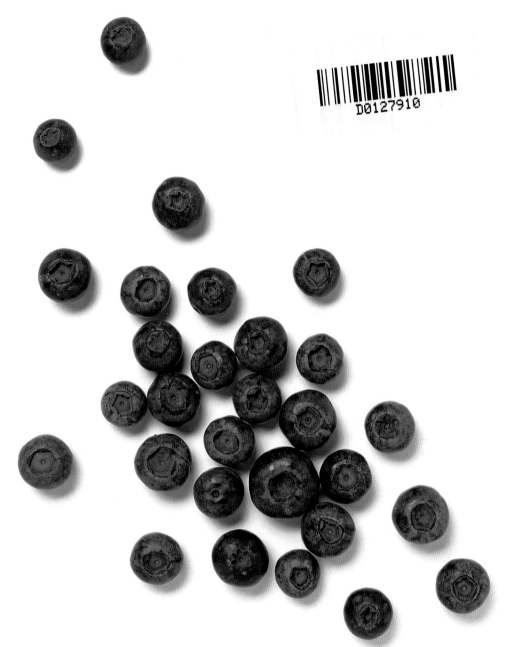

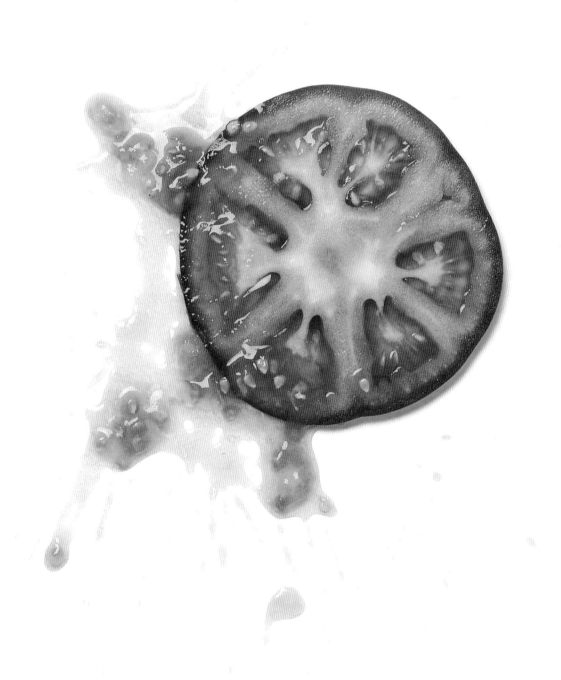

Dr Gillian McKeith's Ultimate Health Plan

The DIET programme that will keep you slim for life

MICHAEL JOSEPH
an imprint of PENGUIN BOOKS

MICHAEL JOSEPH

Published by the Penguin Group
Penguin Books Ltd, 80 Strand, London WC2R ORL, England
Penguin Group (USA) Inc., 375 Hudson Street, New York, New York 10014, USA
Penguin Group (Canada), 90 Eglinton Avenue East, Suite 700, Toronto, Ontario,
Canada M4P 2Y3 (a division of Pearson Penguin Canada Inc.)
Penguin Ireland, 25 St Stephen's Green, Dublin 2, Ireland (a division of Penguin Books Ltd)
Penguin Group (Australia), 250 Camberwell Road,
Camberwell, Victoria 3124, Australia (a division of Pearson Australia Group Pty Ltd)
Penguin Books India Pvt Ltd, 11 Community Centre,
Panchsheel Park, New Delhi – 110 017, India
Penguin Group (NZ), cnr Airborne and Rosedale Roads, Albany,
Auckland 1310, New Zealand (a division of Pearson New Zealand Ltd)
Penguin Books (South Africa) (Pty) Ltd, 24 Sturdee Avenue,
Rosebank, Johannesburg 2196, South Africa

Penguin Books Ltd, Registered Offices: 80 Strand, London WC2R ORL, England

www.penguin.com

First published 2006
4

Text copyright © Dr Gillian McKeith, 2006
Portrait photography copyright © Colin Bell, 2006
Food photography copyright © Benoît Audureau, 2006

The moral right of the author has been asserted

Set in New Clarendon and Trade Gothic
Designed and typeset by Smith & Gilmour, London
Colour Reproduction by Dot Gradations Ltd, UK
Printed in Great Britain by Butler & Tanner Ltd, Frome, Somerset

A CIP catalogue record for this book is available from the British Library

ISBN-13: 978-0-718-14891-1
ISBN-10: 0-718-14891-6

Every effort has been made to ensure that the information in this book is accurate. The
information in this book will be relevant to the majority of people but may not be applicable
in each individual case so it is advised that professional medical advice is obtained for specific
information on personal health matters. Neither the publisher not the author accept any legal
responsibility for any personal injury or other damage or loss arising from the use or misuse
of the information and advice in this book. All vitamin, mineral and herbal supplements are
sold in varying strengths, so always check the dosage on the packaging

CONTENTS

INTRODUCTION

DAY 1: GOING TO NEW HEIGHTS OF ULTIMATE HEALTH

This is the book that will take you to new heights of wellness and new degrees of health on all levels: physically, emotionally and spiritually. We go deeper and further than I have ever done before in any other book. For that to happen I want you to know where I'm coming from. I want you to feel you know me, and more importantly I want you to know yourself better. The following pages are the culmination of years of working with clients, distilled and ready for you to put straight into practice.

To succeed, you will find out how to really look at yourself on all levels: your diet, your lifestyle, your attitude and your emotions. I will share with you some of the very same tools that I use with my clients. This book is a real workbook for you – in essence it's your own consultation.

Before we start, here's a story which just about sums me up! Anyone who knows me knows I am a bit wild about my mango smoothies. I just love them because they're so good for you, I can load them up with superfoods, minerals and vitamins, and they taste so delicious. I start every day with a smoothie.

My brother tells me I'm obsessed, but I just say that I'm passionate about smoothies and your health. It's not that I'm obsessed, but I do now know that achieving ultimate health requires active engagement, passion and determination. We control more about our own health than most people realise. But back to my Smoothie Story . . .

Several years ago, I was asked to be the keynote speaker to a convention of health practitioners and doctors in Sofia, Bulgaria. To prepare myself for the trip, I spent the night before my departure whipping up five separate flasks of mango smoothies. Upon arrival at the extremely nice hotel room in Sofia, I grabbed a smoothie flask. As I made the final twist of the lid, I vaguely felt some kind of a pressure build-up inside the flask. I was just looking forward to my smoothie, but then there was a loud pop as the lid disengaged itself and flew off like a rocket. I have never seen anything quite like it and probably never will again. A thick concoction of four finely blended ripe mangoes, three large bananas and two peaches had exploded all over my hotel room:

the ceiling, the walls, the drapes, the bedding and my clothes were all splattered and covered with mango goo.

I was horrified. You hear this kind of thing about British rock stars or an American heavy metal band trashing their hotel room. But whoever heard of a TV nutritionist from Scotland destroying the place with mango pudding? And then it dawned on me. I looked within myself and realised that for any person to travel almost 2,000 miles from home with five flasks of mango smoothies in tow must be a seriously passionate and determined nutritionist who will go to the end of the earth for ultimate health.

I don't want you to follow in my mango exploding footsteps but this is the kind of determination and passion for health that I want you to embrace. It is already within your grasp; you just need to learn how to unlock it. I will give you the tools to discover your own desires, set your goals and achieve them. This book is like the roadmap; once you know the route, then the rest is easy. Flick the switch and discover the power to eat well, feel well and look fab.

This book shows you the way to manifest a new you, a new body, new foods, new cells, a new attitude and a renewed love and appreciation for yourself, so that your natural energy is free and clear to create ultimate health and happiness. And by the way, if you ever get the wild desire to travel halfway across the world with flasks of pressurised nutrient-infused fruit smoothies ready for an imminent explosion, then just go for it and laugh your head off afterwards.

Wishing you Love & Light,

Gillian

Dr Gillian McKeith (PhD)
www.drgillianmckeith.com
JANUARY 2006

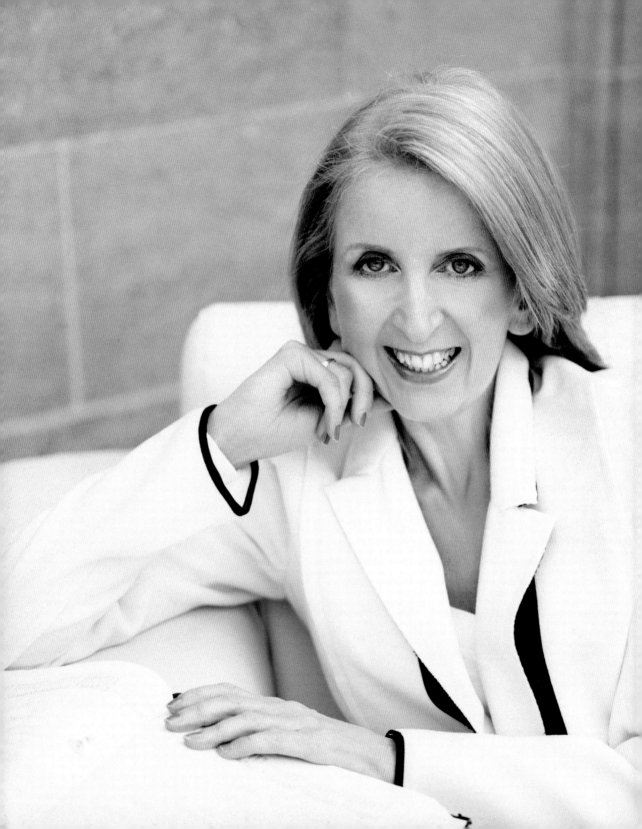

level one
the wake-up call

THE FOOD DIARY

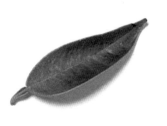

Many people convince themselves that they eat a healthy diet, when the reality is somewhat different. If you think you eat really well, see if this typical exchange between a new client and myself rings any bells. Here's how the play goes:

Gillian: Hi, nice to meet you.
Client: Hello, it's great to be here.
Gillian: Let's talk about your food. Do you eat well?
Client: Pretty well.
Gillian: And how do you feel?
Client: I'm bloated, tired and I just don't seem to have much energy. I get jittery, suffer from headaches, sweet cravings, mood swings, stress and insomnia. I just don't feel very healthy.
Gillian: Well, how would you evaluate your food intake?
Client: I think it's okay. Like everybody, I have my blips now and again.
Gillian: Give me an example of a blip.
Client: I like chocolate now and again.
Gillian: How much chocolate?
Client: Just a little piece of chocolate each day.
Gillian: Let's cut out the dance here. Be straight with me. I need to know, how many *bars* of chocolate are you eating each day?
Client: On average two, unless I feel really ratty, then it might be more, especially during my period.
Gillian: Please may I see your Food Diary?
Client: Fine. But it's not been a typical week. I really don't eat that much chocolate. This week was an exception. Really!

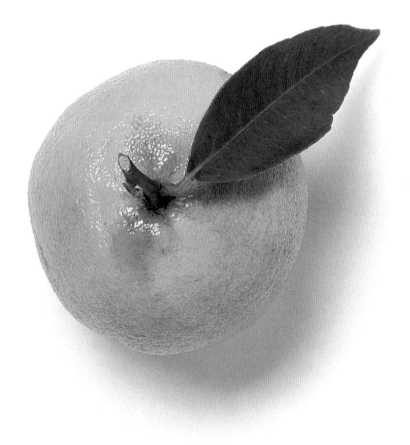

I look at the Food Diary and I am shocked by the sheer number of chocolate bars that this woman is eating on a regular, daily basis. No wonder she's suffering. But she's taken the all-important first step towards making a positive change and she'll soon know how good it feels to leave those headaches and cravings behind.

My point here is to illustrate that many people, when they meet me for the first time, tell me that they eat a good, healthy diet. Most think or say they eat healthy foods, almost like a trained, autopilot response. In reality though, when I start to delve further I often find that it is not so healthy after all, and then I get to the honest truth. There is often very little correlation between the first utterance of 'I eat healthily' to the practical reality.

Seven Day Diary

For the next seven days, I want you to get real, be honest with yourself and write down in a notebook everything you eat and drink. And I mean *absolutely every morsel*. Do not exclude anything. This food and beverage diary exercise will help you make conscious rather than automated choices about the food you eat. Most unhealthy eating is a mindless, habitual, conditioned reaction to a wide variety of cues, few of which have to do with hunger. By writing down what you're doing, when you're doing it, and how you're feeling at the time, you will give yourself the opportunity to transform a habit into a conscious choice. It will help you to identify your goals and how you're going to achieve them.

A complete picture of you and your diet will open a window and give you an understanding of your eating habits and their effect on your life, energy levels, weight and health. So, from the minute you get up until the minute you go to bed, I want you to document everything. It may seem like a pain at first, but once you get going you will soon get into the swing.

No Half Measures

No half measures here now. If you have
a bar of chocolate every night, write that
down. Excluding the chocolate from the
list does not mean that you did not eat it!
Include times of eating and drinking,
quantities, brand names and how the food
is prepared – fried, steamed, grilled, baked
– and whether or not the food is made from
scratch, is fresh, packaged, microwaved or
raw/not cooked. Be as specific as possible,
so even include the amount of sugar you
add to tea, whether or not the tea is herbal
or regular, if you add salt to your cooking,
the amount of water you drink and
whether it is fizzy or still. The more detail,
the more complete the picture of you.

Exercise

I also want you to take note of all the
exercise you take, from walking to work
through to a full gym workout. Note down
the time, what type of exercise and
how long.

Sleep

Keep a note of your sleep patterns. What
time do you go to bed? How long does it
take to fall asleep and how many unbroken
hours of sleep do you have? Do you wake
up energized or exhausted?

Food and Mood

Last but not least, note how you feel before
eating a meal, a snack, any food or drink.
You may feel energized, tired, itchy, or just
fine. Write down how you feel afterwards,
only if you notice a difference. You may not
experience any change and that is okay.
Your feeling may be positive or negative.
Write it down. Here are some guidelines
to help:

1. How hungry do you feel before food?
Are you hungry after food?
2. How do you feel physically? For example,
do you feel headachy, shaky or tired?
You may feel just fine, so do not make
any comment.
3. How do you feel emotionally? For
example, do you feel stressed, bored,
apathetic, happy? Are you upset about
something while eating? Did you have
an argument with someone before eating?
4. Observe how you feel afterwards, if you
notice a change. Are you satisfied or still
hungry? Are there any emotional feelings
or physical changes? Are you sleepy, tired,
energized? Don't go looking for something
that is not there. Simply take note if you
notice a physical feeling or emotion.

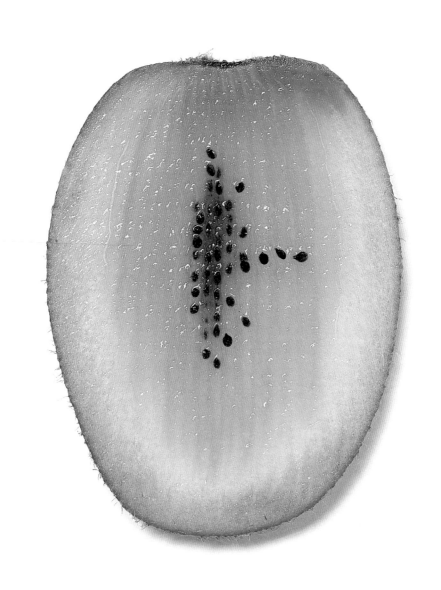

Dr Gillian McKeith's dietary intake form

I promise to be 100 per cent honest, truthful and exact about everything I eat and drink over the next seven days.

Signature ....

1. Time of day
2. Food and beverage intake in detail to include quantities and brands if appropriate
3. How the food is prepared
4. Where and with whom the food is eaten
5. Moods/emotions

EXAMPLE DAY

Friday

7am Cup of tea. Slept badly, dreamt I was late for everything. Feel tired.
8am Hazelnut yoghurt, 150g, made with added cream and sugar.
10am Bottle of water.
1pm Chicken salad sandwich, no mayo. Small bag ready salted crisps. Apple.
1.30pm Cup of tea.
3pm Feel tired and fed up. Chocolate bar.
4pm Glass of water and cup of peppermint tea.
7pm Glass of wine with handful of olives.
8pm Dinner: swordfish and veggies, followed by lemon tart with fresh raspberries . . . washed down with another 2 glasses of wine.
11pm Cup of tea, then bed.

THE COLLECTOR

I had a client once who was an investment banker. A confessed workaholic, he grafted all hours and rarely left his office. Breakfast, lunch and even dinner were eaten at his desk while he was talking on the phone and doing the big deals. When he made an appointment with me, I asked him to bring the wrappers of everything he ate and drank for a week. When he arrived, he lugged into my office a huge bin bag, bursting at the seams, packed with a week's worth of what he had scoffed.

As we looked through the wreckage it was clear he had not eaten anything real for that entire week. Tumbling on to my desk came wrapper after wrapper from chocolate bars, sweets, chewing gum, sugary drinks – dozens of them – and a few greasy takeaway wrappers. He was living on sweets.

We both surveyed the mountain of paper and plastic. Mr Banker blurted out, 'I know this cannot be good for me but I have no clue what to do about it. I am too damn busy.'

Excuse number one had hit his lips. The excuse I hear all the time. Too busy for what? Too busy to eat? Too busy to care? Too busy to live?

It turned out that the banker had been told by his doctor that he was a walking time bomb, heading for Type II Diabetes. He was exhausted all the time, three stones overweight, plagued with headaches and making costly mistakes at work. This moment of realization was the first step in his transformation to wellness: the glaring recognition for the first time of the cocktail of non-foods, chemicals, additives and rubbish that he was forcing his body to exist on.

The Collector in You

In addition to your Food Diary I want you to become a packaging collector this week. Keep all the packaging from everything that you eat and drink, healthy or unhealthy, for seven days. Put it all in a large box or a bag.

So, if you have a microwaveable ready meal on Tuesday night, I want you to keep the packaging with the ingredients listing. The same goes for a takeaway, hold on to all the bags and cartons that come with it. If you use ingredients to make something fresh, make a note of where the ingredients come from. For example, if you eat three fresh carrots write this information on a piece of paper and add it to the bag with all the bottles, packets and so on. If the carrots were organic, mark that information down too. By the end of seven days you may have quite a collection.

Why Am I Collecting?

1. To get in touch with exactly what you put into your body
2. To learn to read food labels
3. To start evaluating what is in the food that you are eating
4. To see just how much fresh food you are consuming versus processed

THE RECKONING

At the end of the seven days, I want you to sit down in front of all of your packaging and take a good look through. You might be surprised or even horrified. This is a brilliant visual exercise for waking up to the reality of your diet.

GET INTO LABELS

The food label is a reliable, accurate, user-friendly source of valuable nutritional information. What you learn from reading and comparing food labels will help you to avoid ingredients and additives that may not be good for you. Knowledge leads to empowerment and better choices.

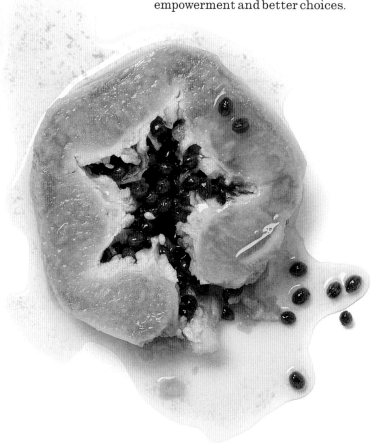

How Do I Read the Ingredients List?

The ingredients are listed in descending order by weight and include any colour additives, preservatives, nutrients, fats or sugars that have been added. So if a packet of food has sugar as the first ingredient, then you know that the sugar content within that food is high.

What About Food Additives?

There are over 14,000 man-made chemicals added to our food supply today. Our bodies are not designed to break down and digest so many chemicals and food additives. Be aware of the types of chemicals and food additives you are consuming. Some additives in our food have been linked to a variety of health problems including headaches, fatigue and allergies.

TOP 10 FOOD ADDITIVES TO AVOID

- ► Acesulfame-K
- ► Artificial colourings
- ► Aspartame
- ► BHA & BHT
- ► Caffeine
- ► Monosodium Glutamate (MSG)
- ► Nitrite and Nitrate
- ► Potassium Bromate
- ► Sulfites
- ► Tartrazine

If you need a dictionary to decipher the label, chances are you should not be eating that food.

Food Claims

Claims are sometimes made on food packaging such as 'low in fat and cholesterol' or 'fortified with iron'. Here's a quick guide to some of the problems associated with these claims.

WHAT IS FORTIFIED?

Fortified means that a nutrient that is not naturally present in a food has been added. Natural foods contain an abundance of nutrients that are instantly recognizable to the human body and so easily digested. The thousands of nutrients and phytochemicals found in natural foods work in perfect harmony with each other. Fortified foods tend to contain isolated nutrients that have been shown to be commonly deficient in our diet. The problem is that the natural synergy of the nutrients is lost when they are taken separately like this.

Foods fortified with calcium are one example. The type of calcium used is often calcium carbonate, which is poorly utilized and can lead to a build up of calcium deposits that can actually cause health problems. Calcium utilization is affected by magnesium, vitamin D, boron, fibre and the ratio of other minerals to the calcium. All of these are likely to be out of balance if calcium is added to a food. It's not the way nature intended it.

WHAT IS ENRICHED?

Rice is a good example. Everybody tells me how much they love white rice. But the difference between brown rice and white rice is not just in colour. The milling and polishing that converts brown rice into white rice destroys approximately two thirds of the vitamin B3, 80 per cent of the vitamin B1, 90 per cent of the vitamin B6, plus half of the manganese, half of the phosphorus, 60 per cent of the iron, and all of the dietary fibre and essential fatty acids. The resulting white rice is simply a refined starch that is largely bereft of its original health-boosting nutrients. You'll probably find that white rice has been 'enriched' with vitamins B1, B3, and iron. But the form of these nutrients when added back into the processed rice is not the same as in the original unprocessed version, and at least 11 lost nutrients are not replaced at all.

Keep Them Low

On the nutrition label, the nutrients that most people eat too much of are listed first. It is a good idea to read the labels and choose foods that are low in the following:

- Salt
- Sugar
- Saturated fat

Salt

Salt is needed by the body to help cells take up nutrients and balance fluid levels, but it is only needed in tiny amounts. The recommended limit of salt is 6g per day. Salt is hidden in so many foods, even before you shake it on your food. Try to make sure you eat 'no added salt' foods as much as possible and instead of adding salt when cooking, add flavour through dried and fresh herbs.

When reading nutrition labels also watch out for 'sodium', as 1g of sodium is roughly equivalent to 2.5g salt. Table salt is 40 per cent sodium and I want you to cut out using table salt completely. Too much salt can raise your blood pressure, which in turn can lead to heart disease, stroke or kidney problems.

Sugar Junkies

Sugars are a type of carbohydrate that occurs naturally in foods such as fruits. Added sugars are those that do not occur naturally in a food but are added during processing or preparation. Foods containing added sugars provide calories but may have few vitamins and minerals. Frequently consumed foods with added sugars include soft drinks, cakes, biscuits, pies, ice cream, sweets, chocolate, many ready meals and some tinned foods. Consuming too many of these foods may cause weight gain or prevent you from eating more nutritious foods.

Because added sugars are not always called 'sugar', it can be difficult to identify them in food. Following is a list of just some of the names for added sugars. If one of these names appears first or second in the ingredients list, the food is probably high in added sugar.

- Brown sugar
- Cane juice
- Corn sweetener
- Corn syrup
- Dextrose
- Fructose
- Glucose
- High-fructose
- Invert sugar
- Lactose
- Maltose
- Raw cane sugar
- Raw sugar
- Sucrose syrup

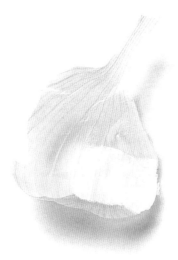

The Fat Problem

Some fats are very good for you, in fact they are essential, hence their name, 'essential fatty acids'. Most labels won't say if the total fat content is good or bad fat, so I would urge you to get your good fat intake from avocados, seeds, nuts and fish.

BAD FAT FOOD is difficult to digest and can lead to weight gain. Saturated fat, which often is included on the nutrition breakdown, is known to raise levels of cholesterol and increase the risk of heart disease, so always watch out for that if it is listed.

SATURATED FATS are solid at room temperature (butter, lard) and found mainly in animal produce and dairy products, in hard and soft margarines, cooking fats, cakes, biscuits, savoury snacks and other processed foods, confectionery and chocolate.

TRANS FATS – the evil twin of saturated fats – are produced when vegetable and fish oils are hydrogenated to turn them into margarine or shortening. Like saturated fats from animal food, they block the conversion of essential fats, and research has shown that they may be even worse for you than saturated fats as they not only raise levels of bad blood cholesterol but also lower levels of good. Low fat spreads often contain hydrogenated or partially hydrogenated fats.

Also be aware that LOW FAT FOODS often contain sugar to make up for the lack of flavour from the fats. If sugar is not used by the body for energy it can be converted into fat and stored just like fat, so there's no benefit to be gained from swapping to 'low fat' if it simply means high sugar.

YOUR DIET PROFILE

Take your Food Diary and the packaging you have collected and create your own individual diet profile by following these simple steps. Evaluate the current reality and then write down how you'd like to improve each aspect of your diet, i.e. your goals.

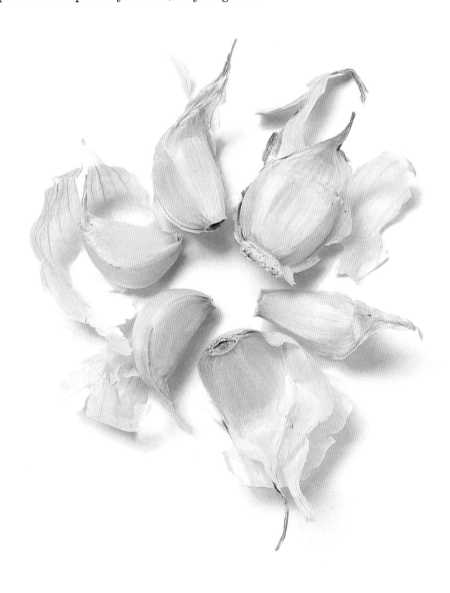

1 PERCENTAGE OF FRESH FOOD VERSUS NON-FRESH

The first thing I want you to look at is the amount of fresh food you eat versus non-fresh. Is it about half and half, or more like 75 per cent processed and 25 per cent fresh? If you can eat a few more meals that are from fresh ingredients, then that would be a good change to make. Processed and refined foods are typically high in sugar, salt, saturated fat, trans fats, chemicals, additives and preservatives, and low in nutrients. All these substances simply aren't good for you. By contrast, healthy fresh food is rich in the nutrients you need.

2 ARE YOU EATING YOUR FIVE PORTIONS OF VEGETABLES A DAY?

Vegetables are nutritional superstars. They are powerful sources of health- and immune-boosting antioxidants, vitamins, minerals and phytochemicals which not only help you look and feel good, but also offer vital protection against all kinds of disorders and reduce the risk of diabetes, heart disease and cancer. Vegetables also aid digestion and encourage the elimination of toxins and waste because of their fibre content. The question is, are you getting enough of them?

3 ARE YOU EATING THE SAME THINGS EVERY DAY?

When I see a Food Diary for the first time, one of the main things that strikes me is the lack of variety. Often people eat the same things every day, day in, day out. Even if you are eating a healthy food, you should not eat the same thing every single day. So if you like porridge oats, do not eat them seven mornings a week. It is easy to develop food sensitivities when you expose your body to the same food all the time. If you can, eat foods on a four-day rotation. So if you have porridge on a Monday, don't eat it again until Thursday.

4 ARE YOU JUNKING OUT?

How many takeaways, ready meals or processed foods are you eating? Many are loaded with salt, sugar, colourings, additives, hardened (partially hydrogenated or hydrogenated) vegetable oil and other hidden evils. Plus many of the good nutrients are processed out of these foods, so if you live on them you will literally be malnourished. Stop eating them. Junk foods are a direct assault on your body, increasing its toxic load and promoting obesity, heart disease and other health problems.

5 ARE YOU A SUGAR JUNKIE?

Are you consuming sugar at breakfast, lunch, dinner, in your teas and coffees? Is it hidden in your cereal boxes and are you adding more? Are you a fizzy drink fanatic? You must limit your intake of sugar, sweeteners and sugary foods if you want to feel well and lose weight. Table sugar contains nothing more than empty calories and goes straight into your blood stream. It causes rapid swings in blood sugar and energy levels. Natural sweeteners like fruit juice or fresh fruits are the best alternatives.

6 ARE YOU A SALT JUNKIE?

Too much salt in your diet may upset the sodium/potassium balance in your body and trigger high blood pressure and heart disease. Salty diets are also linked to fluid retention and kidney stones. The main sources of sodium in your diet are table salt, cooking salt, sauces and processed foods. It's hidden in so many things. Steer clear of salty crisps, cured and smoked meats. Instead of adding salt to boost flavour, experiment with herbs and spices for alternatives. If you do use a very small amount of salt then be sure to use sea salt.

7 DO YOU EAT ENOUGH RAW FRUITS AND VEGETABLES?

It is important to eat raw food every day. You will feel so much better if you increase your intake of raw foods. Are you eating raw foods as part of every meal? If not, then there's room for improvement! To include more raw in your diet:

► Make raw fruit smoothies in the mornings.
► Eat fruit salads.
► Snack on fruits.
► Include sprouted seeds like alfalfa sprouts in your salads.
► Every time you eat something cooked, always include some raw leaves, vegetables or salad.
► In the colder months, when you may be eating more soups and stews, toss in lots of raw herbs and even raw veggies just before serving.
► In the warmer months, eat more raw foods. At least half your main meal should be raw.

8 IS THERE TOO MUCH WHEAT IN YOUR DIET?

Are you eating toast for breakfast every day, snacking on sandwiches, eating bread with dinner and toast for supper? Wheat contains gluten, which can lead to digestive problems in some and may interfere with metabolism in others. If you want to lose weight, you will have to go wheat-free for a while. And as part of a healthy, varied diet it's important to introduce other grains such as brown rice, barley, spelt, millet, amaranth, quinoa and rye.

9 ARE YOU DRINKING ENOUGH WATER?

Your body is made up of two thirds water, so water intake and distribution is vital for balancing hormones, eliminating waste products, keeping your cells working and delivering nutrients to your organs. Dehydration is a sure way to help yourself put on weight. You need to drink at least six to eight glasses of water each day.

10 DO YOU EAT TOO MANY 'WHITE' FOODS?

White pasta, white rice and white bread are refined foods. They are not only low in nutrients but quick to release sugar. This means you may get a quick high followed by long slumps of energy. Cut them out.

11 COMPARE YOUR INTAKE OF GOOD FATS V BAD FATS

You should try to obtain as little fat as possible from saturated fats or trans fats found in animal products and processed foods and as much as possible in the form of essential fatty acids, particularly omega 3 and 6. Without sufficient quantities of EFAs your body cannot manufacture the hormones and chemicals you need to stay healthy, happy and trim. So, in a nutshell, are you eating enough avocados, oily fish, olive oil, hemp oil, seeds and nuts?

12 DO YOU USE HERBS AND SPICES?

Gentle spices and herbs add taste and variety to your food and most have health benefits too. It's time to ditch the salt and pepper and be adventurous.

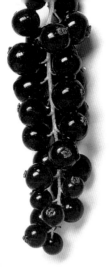
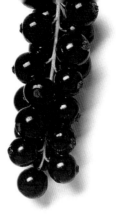
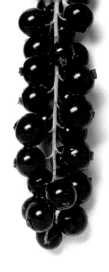

13 ARE YOU A CAFFEINE ADDICT?

Caffeine contains a chemical called benzoic acid which has a
toxic and dehydrating effect on your body. Caffeine in tea, coffee,
chocolate and caffeinated soft drinks also acts as a stimulant and
causes a fast rise in blood pressure and blood sugar, followed by
a quick drop which contributes to a roller coaster ride of mood
swings, fatigue, concentration problems, headaches and anxiety.
To top it all off, caffeine whips your adrenal glands into exhaustion
causing an imbalance in stress hormones. Poor adrenal function
leaves you prone to putting on pounds around your middle, and it
leaves you feeling wiped out. So, far from being a quick pick-me-up,
caffeine just makes you feel tired, irritable, incontinent and old
before your time. Try caffeine-free herb teas instead.

14 ARE YOU EATING ORGANICALLY?

If you want to reduce the toxic load on your body, organic food
is really the best way forward. The production of organic food
is governed by strict standards and the use of chemicals and
preservatives is avoided. Many supermarkets now sell organic
food but if you can't find or afford much organic food remember
than even if you eat organic food now and again or just stick to
organic fruit and veg it can still help to enhance your health.

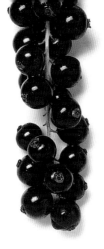
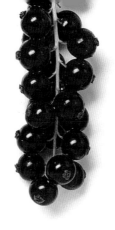
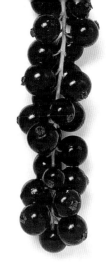

15 HOW MUCH RED MEAT DO YOU EAT?

How often are you eating red meat? A diet heavy in high protein,
fatty, red meat can be hard going on your digestion. It can deplete
nutrients, overwork the kidneys and liver, cause digestive problems
and increase the proportion of harmful bacteria that live in your
gut. Several studies link too much red meat to kidney stones, colon
disorders, heart disease and constipation. There is no red meat
on my *Ultimate Health Plan* because I want to get your digestive
system back in top working order. But this doesn't mean you can
never eat red meat again. Personally, I don't eat meat, but if you
want to make it an occasional food, that's fine. If you do, then make
sure to buy organic, quality, lean and trimmed meat and eat with
lightly steamed green veg and a salad of leaves and sprouted seeds.

16 WHERE ARE YOU EATING?

If you eat out a lot, are you choosing restaurants with good,
healthy, quality foods? Are you making healthy choices when
ordering? For example, opting for grilled fish instead of fried,
side vegetables instead of chips?

17 ARE YOU A NON-VEGGIE-EATING VEGETARIAN?

Removing meat from your diet and surviving on cheese sandwiches, crisps and beans-on-white-toast is not going to hack it. I have met many vegetarians over the years who do not eat a balanced diet. They have stopped eating meat but seem to survive on lots of crisps and junk foods. This is not a healthy way to live. If you want to be a vegetarian, you must learn how to do it properly. You need to eat widely from fruits, vegetables, seeds, nuts, beans, grains, legumes, seaweeds, sprouted seeds, sprouted nuts and pulses, and possibly eggs and fish, depending on what kind of veggie you are. When properly planned, vegetarian diets are very healthy and as a group, vegetarians are less likely to develop high blood pressure, diabetes, coronary heart disease or obesity.

18 DO YOU EXERCISE MORE THAN THREE TIMES WEEKLY?

You need to move your bahookee every day. Exercise can boost energy in all kinds of ways. It increases circulation and by so doing helps lower LDL (bad) cholesterol and increase HDL (good) cholesterol.

Exercise:
- Can lower blood sugar levels and promote insulin efficiency – fatigue is a symptom of blood sugar imbalance.
- Keeps bowels working efficiently to eliminate waste products your body doesn't need or want and which can slow you down.
- Boosts immunity which means you are less likely to get ill.
- Burns calories and builds up muscles. The more your muscles build up the speedier your metabolism becomes.
- Encourages a good night's sleep.
- Improves your sex life.
- Boosts mood through the release of brain chemicals called endorphins.

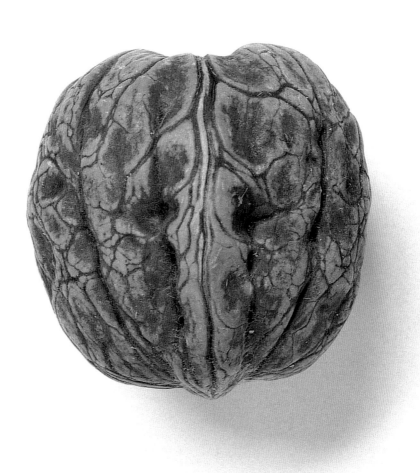

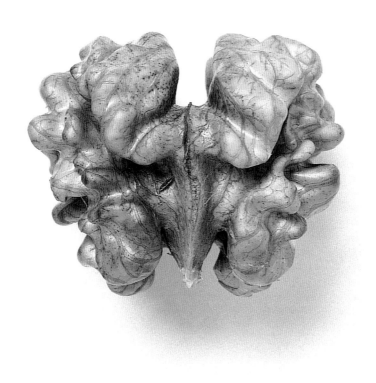

19 ARE YOU SNACKING HEALTHILY AND REGULARLY?

Regular healthy snacking – for example fruit, nuts, seeds
or veggie sticks – is the key to keeping your blood sugar levels
balanced. This means your energy levels stay high and your mood
stays good. It also means that you don't ever feel hungry. If more
than three or four hours is left between meals or snacks you're
more likely to crave unhealthy, high-sugar foods because your
blood sugar levels are low and your stomach is empty.

20 ARE YOU EATING ENOUGH FIBRE A DAY?

Add fibre rich foods to your diet like porridge oats, fruit, seeds,
vegetables, brown rice and beans. Fibre is the bran of the grain,
the cell walls of the vegetables, the pulp of the fruits. In other
words it is the indigestible portion of these foods that improves
intestinal function, helps to grow healthy bacteria in the gut and
helps to prevent disease by ensuring the removal of waste products
and toxins. It also ensures that digestion is healthy and helps
maintain blood sugar balance. Follow my Plan and you'll
automatically get enough.

21 HOW MUCH OF YOUR DIET IS DAIRY?

Dairy products are high in saturated fat which can lead to weight
gain and its associated problems if consumed in high quantities.
I will take you off dairy on my Plan and even afterwards, if you want
to have milk, try goat's milk, sheep's milk or experiment with the
vast array of grain milks such as rice and oat. Cow's milk is
difficult for humans to digest, which is why so many people are
lactose intolerant. Indigestibility can trigger allergic response,
bloating, diarrhoea, flatulence, constipation, PMS, headaches,
irritability, fatigue and weight problems.

22 WHAT DO YOU EAT WHEN?

Missing breakfast and fasting most of the day, then eating a
large dinner in the evening sends your body confusing signals.
First of all, during the day when you are hardly eating, your body
will slow down its metabolic rate to conserve energy. Then when
you do eat in the evening your body is set up to store as much fat
as possible. After eating, you often go to bed so your body has little
time to use up the calories you have just consumed. Eat during
the day when you need the energy, not at night when activity levels
are typically lower. In other words, are you making sure you eat
a hearty breakfast and lunch and reducing your food intake at
the end of the day? If you are eating a big dinner after 8pm, then
expect to feel sluggish in the morning and to gain weight.

23 IS YOUR ENERGY LOW?

To access energy, it's crucial that your diet is rich in the nutrients
your body needs to function optimally. Fatigue is often a symptom
of blood sugar imbalances caused by poor eating habits, poor
nutrient uptake and nutrient deficiencies. And if you are eating
rubbish a lot of the time, you increase your toxic load which
results in even more fatigue.

Energy Crash = Sugar Binges

When you feel low, a natural reaction is to reach for any kind of food
to give you an energy boost. The problem is that, all too often, those
foods are bad fat, junky, sugary, non-foods that give you short-fuse
energy zaps which are quickly followed by energy slumps and,
eventually, weight gain.

24 ARE YOU STRESSING OUT?

Look through your Food Diary. Did you note any of the following?

- ► Salt or sugar cravings
- ► Feeling bloated after eating, or digestive problems
- ► Mid-afternoon energy slump
- ► Constant hunger
- ► Emotional roller coaster, e.g. depressed, short fuse, anxious, crying, impatient, lack of concentration
- ► Insomnia or difficulty falling asleep
- ► Can't get out of bed in the morning

Is stress making you fat? When you get stressed, your adrenal glands prompt the release of sugar stores into the bloodstream. If stress is prolonged, this sugar stays in your bloodstream, increasing the risk of blood sugar problems that can trigger weight gain. That's without eating anything sugary or fattening!

Think about how you live your life and what kinds of changes you could make to bring about balance. Is most of your life devoted to work related activities? Are you exercising enough to sweat out your stress hormones? And getting some fun in your life is key to a healthy lifestyle.

25 ARE YOU DRINKING TOO MUCH ALCOHOL?

Alcohol stimulates your appetite and weakens your liver (your body's fat burning powerhouse) and is full of sugar. The odd glass of wine here or there won't hurt, but if weight loss is your goal, forget about it until you reach your desired weight. It will be worth it.

Example goals

- ► I want to be slim

- ► I want to banish my daily headaches

- ► I want to wake up with energy

- ► I want to sleep peacefully through the night

- ► I want brighter eyes

- ► I want radiant skin

- ► I want to feel more relaxed

- ► I want to be more energized in the afternoon

- ► I want to stop slumping in front of the TV every night

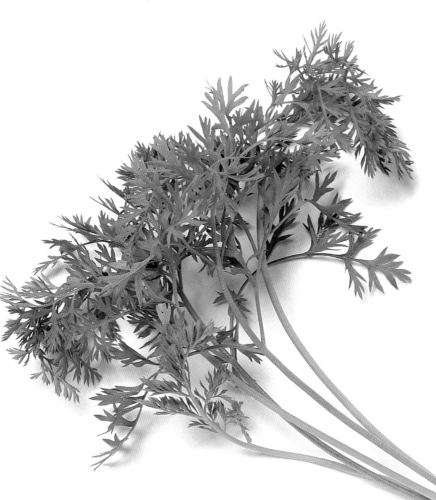

I want to stop eating junk
and start eating fresh, natural
foods full of goodness!

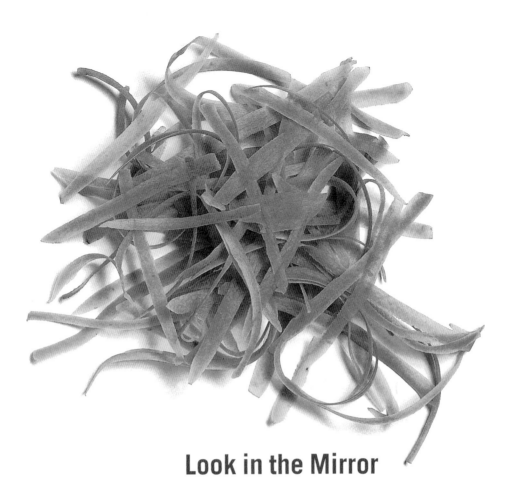

Look in the Mirror

The other morning, I got my children to school late because I needed to have a very long, drawn out consultation to help the babysitter with something. As I was finally going out of the door to work, my Mum called and said she absolutely had to talk to me that minute and it could not wait. Just as I managed to hang up, a friend called. She had just had a row with her partner and needed a shoulder to cry on. I arrived at work late for a meeting, full of all the excuses of the day, blaming the babysitter, my mother and my friend. I started to justify, 'If somebody calls me then how can I get to my next place on time?' A colleague observed that I needed boundaries and discipline and not excuses. Suddenly I realized I was blaming Mum, friend and babysitter for my being Miss Tardy, and that just wasn't good enough.

When consulting with clients, the number of excuses for not eating properly is beyond a joke:

▶ My boyfriend likes pub grub.
▶ My girlfriend eats like a sparrow so there is nothing to eat in the fridge.
▶ My husband hates the taste of health food.
▶ My kids won't eat any of it.
▶ I don't have the time to do what you want, Gillian.
▶ It's all too expensive.

It is so easy to think of excuses. It's much harder to take responsibility for yourself.

▶ Stop blaming others for all the problems in your life.
▶ Stop blaming the fact that you have to go to work for having no time to prepare your food.
▶ Stop blaming your parents for your being overweight.
▶ Stop blaming your husband for influencing your salt intake on the evening meals.
▶ Stop blaming the kids for your chocolate addiction.
▶ Just stop the Blame Game and start taking responsibility, now!

Visualizing your goals

Everything in life is about energy. Some types of energy are more obvious than other types of energy, for example electricity or radio waves. I am a great believer in the power of our own mental energy. Our thoughts and our written or spoken words and messages to ourselves are the keys to achieving our life dreams and this invisible energy should not be underestimated.

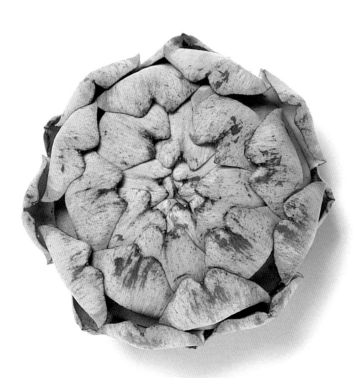
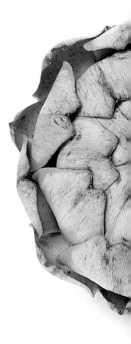

Energy Goal Drawing

Now that you've mapped out your goals, by analysing and evaluating your own food and lifestyle habits and deciding what you want to change, I want you to follow my Energy Goal Drawing Exercise. I want to teach you how to harness energy and make your goals happen. You are literally going to visualize success and reach your potential.

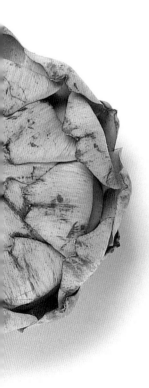

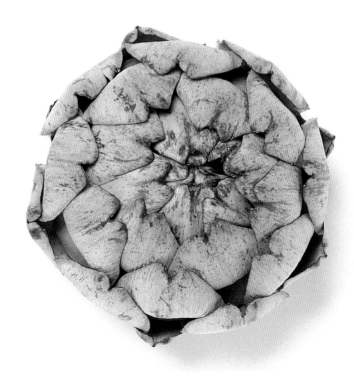

1 START WITH A THOUGHT

What do you want? For instance, you may set an objective that you want to be slimmer, or have more energy or a radiant complexion.

EXAMPLE:

I WANT TO BE SLIMMER

2 WRITE DOWN YOUR THOUGHT

Once you commit your thought to paper with pen, you elevate the thought to a new level of energy.

EXAMPLE:

I AM SLIM

3 ASSESS THE ACTION NEEDED TO ACHIEVE YOUR GOAL

Think about what it will take to become slim, healthy or energized. Break it down into steps. For example, if your goal is to be slim, then your first Action Step is to keep a diary of everything you eat and drink for a week. Your second Action Step might be to throw away all the rubbish foods that I tell you are too nasty for your body. And so on.

EXAMPLE:

STEP 1. Create a Food Diary

STEP 2. Throw out all the rubbishy food

THIS IS ONLY AN EXAMPLE TO ILLUSTRATE THE POSSIBILITIES. I WANT YOU TO PLAN THIS OUT WITH YOUR INDIVIDUAL GOALS AND STEPS TO MATCH. BE CREATIVE AND DO ANYTHING HERE THAT MEETS YOUR OWN ASPIRATIONS.

4 DRAW YOUR GOAL IN A PICTURE

With a black pen, I want you to draw on plain, white paper whatever it is that you want to achieve or how you want to see yourself. So using the slim example, draw a simple figure of yourself looking slim and happy. You do not need to be Rembrandt. All you need to do is draw with stick figures. Put a caption underneath your drawing.

EXAMPLE:

(Your name) IS SLIM. I AM SLIM.

5 DRAW YOUR ACTION STEPS

With a black pen on white paper, draw pictures of you actually going through your Action Steps to reach your end goal.

EXAMPLE:

- A picture of a Food Diary with caption, '(Your name) fills out Food Diary.'
- Complete the pictures and flow it through until you get to your end result and you are now slim.
- Our thoughts have powerful energy. When we write down these thoughts, and even transfer them into pictures, we dramatically intensify them. You are now harnessing the thought into action.
- You can make anything happen. You become the creator of your own destiny.
- Review your drawings every day and redraw them once a month.
- You may find that, on reflection, you wish to elaborate some steps or shorten some steps. After all, you now know that you are the creator of your own destiny.

PLEASE NOTE THAT THE EXAMPLES ABOVE ARE ALL IN THE PRESENT TENSE, WHICH FURTHER STRENGTHENS THE ENERGY OF YOUR THOUGHT. SO INSTEAD OF 'I WILL BE SLIM' IT'S 'I AM SLIM'. THIS METHOD LEAVES NO ROOM FOR DOUBT. WHEN YOU STATE 'I AM' THERE IS NOWHERE ELSE TO GO BUT GET RESULTS AND ACHIEVE SUCCESS.

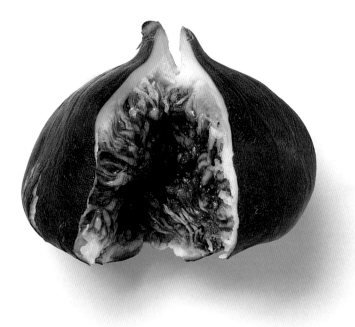

EMBRACING CHANGE

After consulting with hundreds of clients over many years, the greatest challenge I have faced as a nutritionist has been to remove the barriers that most people erect for themselves. We impede our own abilities to fly. We create blockages, doubts, clouded perceptions and negativity every day for ourselves that need not be.

As a practitioner, this is a real problem for me. It can be extremely difficult to tempt a closed soul to the magnificence of new foods and a new lifestyle.

EMBRACE YOUR NEW LIFESTYLE

A plethora of new research now definitively confirms that emotions and physiology are intricately linked and strongly dependent upon each other. We cannot ignore one or the other: the physical and the emotional are both essential to a healthy lifestyle.

In order to be more receptive and emanate an attitude of openness toward change of lifestyle, thus accepting an abundance of new foods, do the following exercise once or twice daily, first thing in the morning and again in the evening:

1. Sit squarely on a firm chair with feet planted on the floor; feel your feet touching the ground.

2. Count up from 1 to 10, closing your eyes and just relax.

3. With eyes closed, listen to the gentle sound of your breath.

4. Breathe through your nose. As you slowly inhale, imagine that you are filling your whole body internally with oxygen, from your toes to the top of your head.

5. Take long slow exhales. Repeat for a couple of minutes, imagining the oxygen flowing through all the cells of your body.

6. Then bring both hands up to your chest, and hold your palms flat on to the chest. Feel your palms against your chest as you breathe. Sit like this for a couple of minutes.

7. You may then place your hands by your side, and say the following, silently to yourself or softly aloud, three times very slowly:

'I open myself to enjoy a whole new array of foods.'

8. Once you have finished saying the above sentence to yourself, then begin to count down from 10 to 1 and slowly open your eyes.

EXCUSE PROMISE

Get a notepad and make a list of the reasons you have used in the past to stop you from improving your health, eating habits and lifestyle choices. Identify routines, habits or lifestyle choices that you have used as a reason for not making positive changes in your life. Here are some of the excuses I have heard over the years:

► **Stressful lifestyle**
► **Too busy**
► **Partner has unhealthy eating habits**
► **Family too demanding, so no energy for myself**
► **Don't know where to start**
► **Too expensive**

Once you have acknowledged your excuses, write the following sentences on your notepad:

I no longer allow any of the above excuses to stop me from achieving my potential. I am free to do anything if I set my mind to it.

Know that the healthier you keep your body and mind, the easier it will be to cope with a demanding lifestyle. Regardless of how unhealthily a partner eats, you do not have to be a follower of that person's bad habits. If your partner encourages you to eat unhealthily, you need to explain to him or her that you are concerned about your health and need to make changes. But you can never blame anyone else for your situation. You cannot blame your hubby for your chocolate cravings or your junk food habits. If your partner doesn't want to go along with you, then you do it for you. Let them do whatever they do. But do not let anyone hold you back from changing your life for the better. Positive change can fit into any lifestyle, no matter how busy. Identifying your excuse blocks is an important start.

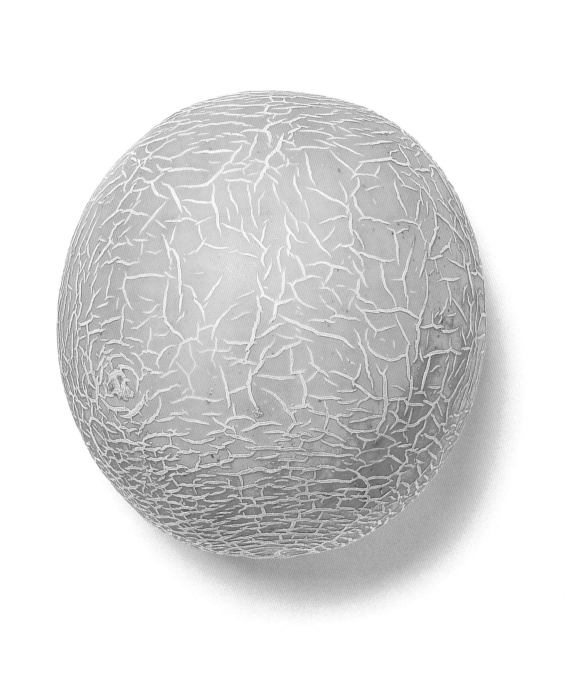

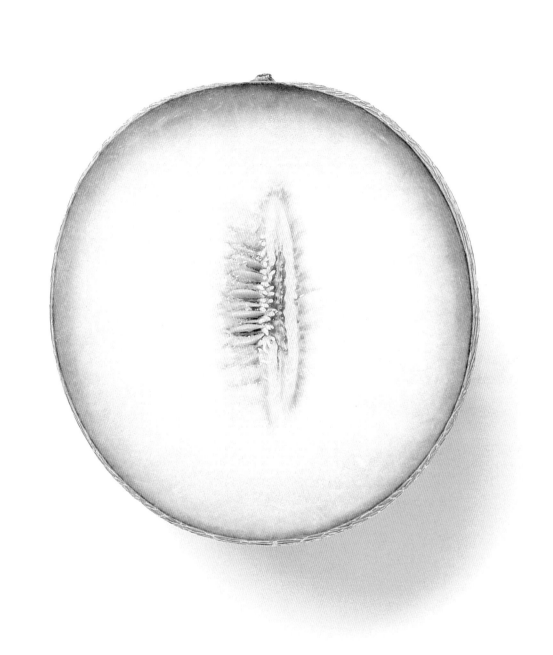

BREAKING BAD HABITS

A habit is something you do repeatedly, over and over. There is no set number of times you need to do something for it to become a habit. It becomes a habit when you do it automatically (without really thinking) and when challenged about the habit, you find it difficult to change. You may even become defensive.

You Are What You Choose

Choice gives you the ability to break bad habits. You always have a choice. You can be a lousy eater and feel dreadful as a result of your poor food choices or you can choose to eat the right foods and realize your health potential.

Magic Bullets

You can create your own magic bullet for change by following the steps outlined on the following pages.

STEP 1 **IDENTIFY YOUR BAD HABITS**

To break bad habits, you need to first of all become aware of what they are. This brings them back into the realm of consciousness and helps you regain your ability to make choices.

Grab a pen and paper and write a list of all the things you do that you know are not good for you, even if you enjoy doing them. For example, eating foods high in sugar and fat, indulging in ice cream, not getting enough exercise, smoking and so on.

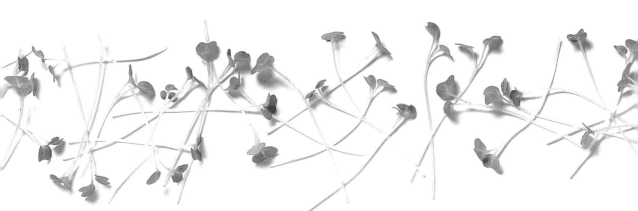

STEP 2 **WHAT'S IN IT FOR YOU?**

What's the motivation for doing something that is bad for you? Why do you do it? Ask yourself why you find this action so compelling. In other words, what's your payoff for doing something that you know isn't good for you? There is always a payoff. But is the payoff worth it? For example, let's say your bad habit is to snack on several bars of chocolate a day. Okay, you get a quick comfort fix when you eat it. But how long does that last? Instead of doing any exercise, you get to slob out in front of the TV. The payoff is probably that you get to unwind and relax. But there are other ways of doing that too.

STEP 3 ARE YOU TRADING OFF?

Analyse the trade off. What is it that you are losing by giving in to your habit? This step should be easier. Why it is that you consider it a bad habit in the first place? Eating too much chocolate is a bad habit because it interferes with your blood sugars and triggers mood swings and it also encourages weight gain. Not exercising enough is a bad habit because it makes you feel unfit and out of shape. In both cases you are trading short-term comfort for long-term weight gain and poor health and wellbeing. When you look at it that way, it doesn't seem like you are making very wise choices, does it? There has to be a better way.

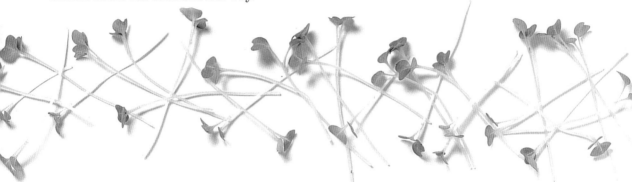

STEP 4 PAYOFF OR TRADE OFF – THAT IS THE QUESTION

Now that you've looked at both sides of the issue – your payoff and your trade off, indulging in a bad habit is no longer an involuntary act. You now know that you are making a choice every time you perform this action. So each time you feel tempted to indulge in a bad habit, remind yourself that you have a choice here. Which do you value more? Do you value more the instant relief you get from snacking unhealthily or slobbing in front of the TV or do you value your overall health and wellbeing more? I want you to become more conscious and aware. Don't go through life unengaged with yourself, mindlessly going through the motions and stuffing rubbish into yourself. If you make conscious choices then you will most likely make the right choices.

If you listen to your body and make intuitive food choices then you will make the right choices.

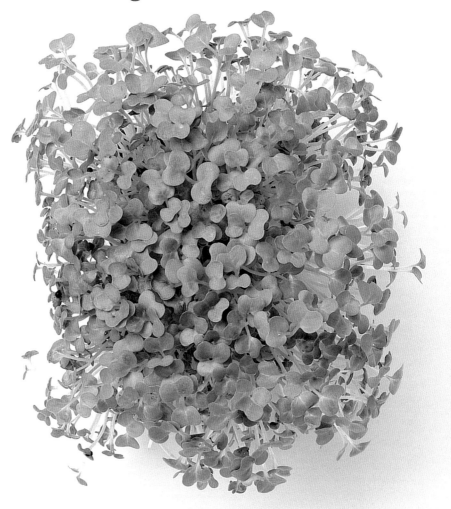

STEP 5 SUBSTITUTING BETTER HABITS

The reason you formed your habits in the first place is that they may have filled a need. Some people say that they needed to feel comforted, so they reached for bad food. Maybe you were feeling tired, so you switched the TV on for the whole evening. I want you to start making active choices to break these old patterns and not fall into the old action. You will be making a choice to perform a better, alternative action in its place. Instead of grabbing a chocolate bar when you feel low, eat an apple or decide to call a friend; write a letter or have a warm bath when you feel tense. Instead of switching the TV on the minute you come in at night, go for a walk. Whatever the new habit is that you substitute is not so relevant. What's important is whether you feel good about the choices you have made. After all, the reason you consider it a bad habit is because it leaves you feeling bad about yourself.

STEP 6 IT'S UP TO YOU

The only way to give bad habits a lifeline is to sink back into denial about why you have bad habits in the first place. Each time you begin to resume your old patterns, the thought will pass through your mind that you are trading one thing for another each time you perform that action. You will be forced to make a choice about continuing your habit. What choices will you make? The one that makes you feel disappointed with yourself or the one that makes you feel positive about yourself? It's up to you. To empower yourself, make the choice that you know intuitively is the right one.

DUMP THE JUNK

This is the scary part when you get to invite Dr Gillian McKeith into your own home. We need to get to the bottom of what's really lurking in your cupboards, have a good clear out and then start afresh.

You have already kept and analysed your Food Diary for seven days, plus inventoried a week's worth of packaging from all that you have eaten.

So now you know what you need to dump, let's get to it! Just in case there is any confusion, here's a checklist of what to clear out for the duration of the Plan:

- **Refined white sugar**
- **Table salt**
- **Processed meats (including bacon, ham, sausages)**
- **Ready meals**
- **Pizzas**
- **Fizzy drinks**
- **Canned foods with added sugar and salt**
- **White bread products**
- **Cakes and biscuits**
- **Packaged foods with added sugar or salt**
- **Crisps**
- **Cow's milk**
- **Cream**
- **Caffeinated drinks (coffee, black tea, colas)**
- **Alcohol (does it help if I tell you that alcohol causes cellulite?)**
- **Hard cheeses**
- **Red meat**
- **Chocolates or chocolate bars**
- **Sweets**
- **Pastries**
- **Ice cream**
- **White rice**
- **White pasta**
- **Margarine and lard**
- **Butter**
- **Wheat products**
- **Hot spicy foods (e.g. chilli sauces)**

Now I know what you are thinking: *There is nothing left to eat!*
Don't be depressed about this list, it looks worse than it really is.

It is a wrench at first, but it's just fantastic that you are
making this change. You are going to eat more foods than you
thought imaginable. There will be so many new choices that you
will be dazzled to the core. It really is a celebration of food which
is going to turn your life around.

It's also worth knowing now that once you make these
changes for a sustained period of time, your body will start to
adjust. In effect, you may even become repelled by the bad food
and actually crave only good foods. Okay, on the surface, you
may think this is a mad Gillian mirage, but I must tell you it
is attainable.

I do not expect you to dump the entire list forever in eternity.
I only demand full compliance for the duration of my Plan, no
questions asked! I'm hoping you'll even enjoy it – just think
of the fresh start.

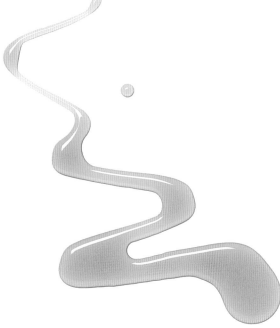

level two
the ultimate health plan

You are now in the thick of it and ready to embark on
my 28 day plan. The good news is that if you need to
lose weight then you will with my new lifestyle. Everyone
knows the results I get. And for even better results,
do my two-day Fat Flush or Detox (Level 3) first.
If you simply want to feel more healthy then my Ultimate
Health Plan will work just as brilliantly for you too.
Whether you want to lose weight or not, YOU ARE NOT
ON A DIET. You have to throw away all previous ideas
about diets. With my programme you are going to eat
more foods than ever before without guilt or denial. And
to get started, all you have to do is follow the Plan day by
day. You do what I tell you and you succeed. It's that
simple. But if you don't, then you lose the game.
You will have to do it my way to the letter of my law.
To repeat: it's my way or the highway. Easy.

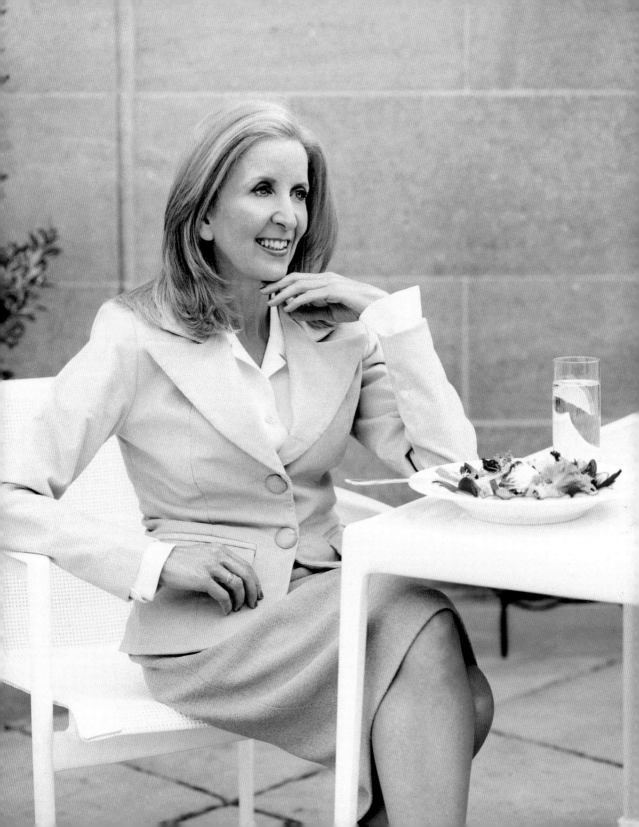

COMPREHENSIVE FOOD LIST

When I look at the first time Food Diaries of new clients who come to me wanting to lose weight, one thing strikes me every single time. They eat more or less the same 10 to 12 foods day in, day out, week in, week out, month in, month out. 'Don't you ever get sick of eating the same foods every single day?' I query. The standard answer is that they don't realize they are eating the same old foods. Bad ones at that.

So, my goal for you is that you tantalize your palate and experience more good, healthy foods than you ever thought possible. Just when you thought there was nothing left to eat, feast your eyes on my list of the best foods to include in your life.

FISH

Carp
Cod
Dover sole
Flounder
Haddock
Hake
Halibut
Herrings
John Dory
Lemon sole
Mackerel
Monkfish
Orange roughy
Pilchards
Plaice
Pollack
Red mullet
Salmon
Sardines
Sea bass
Sea bream
Snapper
Trout
Whitefish

LEAFY GREEN VEGETABLES

Beet greens
Chard
Chicory
Cress
Dandelion flowers
Dandelion greens
Endive
Escarole
Iceberg lettuce
Kale
Lamb's lettuce
Little gem
Loose-leaf lettuce
Mustard greens
Parsley, flat and curly
Rocket
Romaine
Sorrell
Spinach
Swiss chard
Turnip greens
Watercress

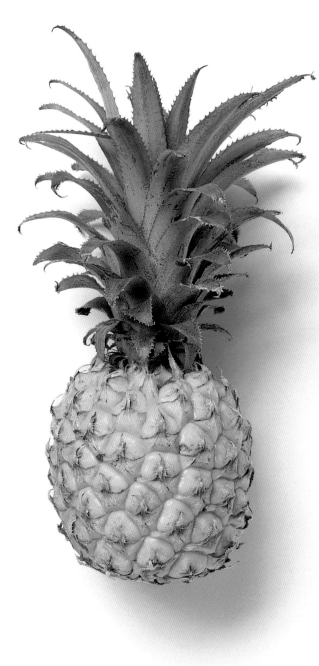

VEGETABLES

Acorn squash
Artichoke
Asparagus
Aubergine
Avocado
Beetroot
Bok choy
Broccoli
Brussels sprouts
Butternut squash
Capsicum
Carrots
Cassava
Chinese leaves
Cauliflower
Celeriac
Celery
Courgettes
Cucumber
Daikon
Fennel
Globe artichoke
Green cabbage
Green peas
Haikido squash
Horseradish
Jerusalem artichoke
Kohlrabi
Leeks

Mangetout
Marrow
Okra
Olives
Onions
Onion squash
Parsnips
Peppers
Purple sprouting
broccoli
Radish
Red cabbage
Salsify
Sauerkraut
Savoy cabbage
Shallots
Shitake mushrooms
Spring onions
Squash
Sugar-snap peas
Swede
Sweetcorn
Sweet potatoes
Tomatoes, yellow,
orange and red
Turnip
White cabbage
Yams

SPROUTS

Beansprouts
Sprouted alfalfa
Sprouted chickpeas
Sprouted clover
Sprouted mung
beans
Sprouted quinoa
Sprouted sunflower
seeds
Any sprouted seed
or nut

BEANS

Adzuki
Black Turtle
Borlotti beans
Broad beans
Butter beans
Cannellini beans
Carob chickpeas
Edamame (steamed
soya beans)
Fava
Flageolet beans
French beans
Garbanzo beans
Great Northern
beans
Green beans
Haricot beans
Lentils, brown and
red
Lima
Mung beans
Navy
Pinto
Runner beans
Soya beans
String beans

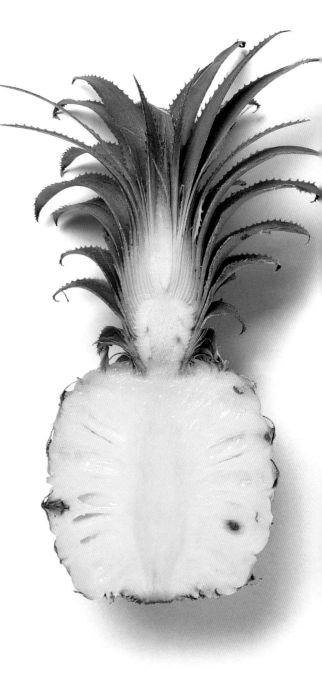

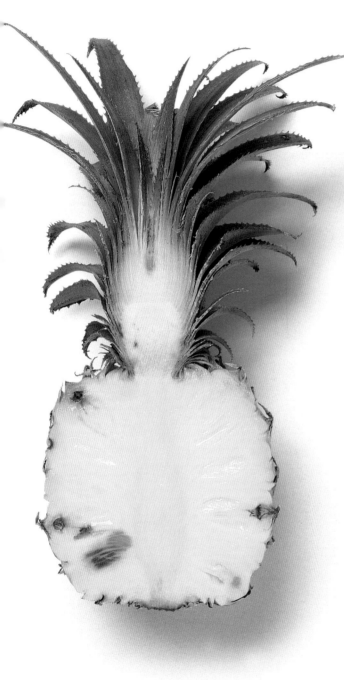

SEEDS

Alfalfa
Flax
Hemp
Poppy
Pumpkin
Sesame
Sunflower

GRAINS

Amaranth
Barley
Basmati rice
Brown rice
Buckwheat
Bulgur wheat
Corn
Kamut
Millet
Oats
Polenta
Quinoa
Red rice
Rye
Spelt
Wild rice

FLOURS

Amaranth flour
Buckwheat flour
Chickpea flour
Gram flour
Lentil flour
Oat flour
Potato flour
Rice flour
Rye flour
Soy flour
Spelt flour
Sunflower seed flour
Tapioca flour
Yellow corn flour

**SEA VEGETABLES
(SEAWEEDS)**

Arame
Dulse
Hijiki
Kelp
Kombu
Nori sea lettuce
Sea palm
Wakame

CONDIMENTS

Brown rice vinegar
Cider vinegar
Miso powder
Miso paste
Mustard
Red wine vinegar
Sauerkraut
Tamari
Umeboshi plum
sauce
Umeboshi vinegar
White wine vinegar

FRESH HERBS +
SPICES (FOR SEASONING)

Agar
All Spice
Aniseed
Basil
Bay leaves
Cardamom
Cayenne
Celery seeds
Chervil
Chives
Cinnamon
Cloves
Coriander
Cumin
Dill
Fenugreek
Garlic

Ginger
Mace
Marjoram
Mint
Mustard seeds
Nutmeg
Oregano
Parsley
Pepper
Rosemary
Saffron
Sage
Star Anise
Tarragon
Thyme
Turmeric
Vanilla pods

RAW NUTS

Almonds
Brazil nuts
Cashew nuts
Chestnuts
Coconut
Filberts
Hazelnuts
Pecans
Pine
Pistachios
Walnuts

FRUIT

Apples
Apricots
Avocados
Bananas
Bilberries
Blackberries
Blackcurrants
Blueberries
Cherries
Cranberries
Currants
Damsons
Dates
Dried fruits
Elderberries
Figs
Gooseberries
Grapefruit, pink and
white
Grapes
Greengages
Guavas
Kiwis
Kumquats
Lemons
Limes
Loganberries
Loquats
Lychees
Mandarins
Mangos
Mulberries

Nashi pears
Nectarines
Papayas
Passion fruit
Paw Paws
Peaches
Pears
Persimmons
Pineapples
Plantains
Plums
Pomegranates
Prickly pears (cactus
fruit)
Prunes
Quince
Raspberries
Redcurrants
Rhubarb
Sharon fruit
Star fruit
Strawberries
Tamarind
Tangerines
Ugli fruit

Melons

Banana melon
Cantaloupe
Galia
Honeydew
Watermelon

SWEETENERS

Agave syrup

Almond extract

Barley malt extract

Brown rice syrup

Carob amazake

Malt extract

Maple syrup

Mirin

Molasses

Vanilla extract

HERBAL TEAS

Borage

Chamomile

Dandelion

Fennel

Ginger

Ginseng

Hawthorn

Horsetail

Lemon balm

Liquorice

Melissa

Nettle

Pau d'arco

Peppermint

Red clover

Red raspberry

Rose hip

Slippery elm

Spearmint

Valerian root

Chicken

Turkey

Tofu

Tempeh

Soya

Yoghurt

DR GILLIAN'S FAVOURITE WEIGHT LOSS FOODS

Adzuki beans

Apples

Avocados

Beet greens

Blueberries

Brown rice

Cardamom

Cucumbers

Dandelion greens

Dandelion tea

Flax seeds

Fruit smoothies

Ginger

Grapes

Leafy greens

Miso soup

Nettle tea

Oats

Oily fish

Papayas

Parsley

Pears

Pink grapefruit

Plums

Quinoa

Raw shelled hemp seeds

Raspberries

Seaweeds: nori, kombu,

wakame, dulse

Soaked almonds

Sprouted seeds: chickpeas,

alfalfa, sunflower seeds,

mung beans, clover

Vegetable juices

Water

Dr Gillian's Food Combo Rules

1. Fruit first, never for dessert.

2. Separate dense proteins from dense carbs at the same meal;
so no chicken and rice together or fish and potatoes together.

Dr Gillian's Top 20 Weight Loss Tips

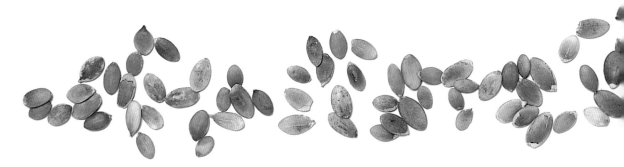

1 EAT MORE, NOT LESS

Eating less than is required to support your basal metabolism will slow your metabolism down. My clients raise metabolism and keep blood sugar levels stable with regular healthy eating. It also helps to prevent bingeing because you never feel famished.

2 SNACKING IS GOOD!

Watch out for the late afternoon and evening slump. If you want to burn fat and prevent your body putting it back on, you must stabilize your blood sugar. In order to do this, you need to eat every two to three hours, which includes healthy snacking mid-morning and mid-afternoon. Fasting, skipping meals, or overly restrictive diets will enable you to lose weight but only in the short term. The weight you primarily lose is water weight and muscle tissue. When you restrict your food intake, your body instinctively thinks it's being starved and shifts into a protective mode by slowing down your metabolism and storing nearly all your calories as body fat. Losing muscle is the last thing you want.

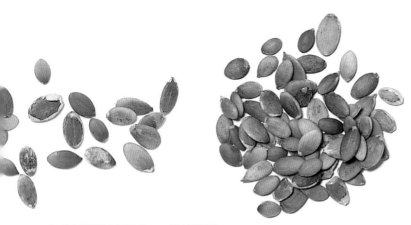

3 DRINK MORE ... WATER

Drink eight glasses of water a day between meals. Have
a large glass of water 20 to 30 minutes before meals. Other
drinks to include are herbal teas and vegetable juices. If you
are exercising you should be drinking even more. Fizzy drinks,
juices, and teas and coffees full of caffeine don't count. Lack
of water can slow the metabolic rate just as lack of food can.
Since water is the body's most important nutrient, the liver
will turn its attention to water retention instead of doing
other duties such as burning fat. Dehydration, because
it causes headaches, lack of concentration and fatigue,
is also often mistaken for hunger.

4 DON'T DRINK TOO MUCH WITH YOUR MEALS

Do not drink copious amounts of liquids with meals, not
even still water. Have a glass of water about half an hour
before you eat and take only little sips during meals if
you must. Fizzy drinks are banned.

5 EAT SOUP FIRST

Have soup before a meal. Studies show that soup before
a meal is a good way to feel satisfied.

6 FIND OUT WHAT'S EATING YOU

Eating foods that aren't healthy can often be triggered by stress, boredom, loneliness, anger, depression and other emotions. Learning to deal with emotions without food is a significant skill that will greatly serve long-term weight control.

7 SLOW DOWN

Eating slowly is one method that can help take off pounds. That's because from the time you begin eating, it takes the brain 20 minutes to start signalling feelings of fullness. Fast eaters often eat beyond their true level of fullness before the 20-minute signal has had a chance to set in. So slow down, take smaller bites and enjoy and savour every tasty morsel. Nutrient uptake is more effective too. When you wolf down your food, you are not able to digest your food nutrients as effectively. Eating too quickly can overload your stomach causing gas and bloating. Also you tend to gulp more air when you eat quickly. So remember to eat regular meals and eat them slowly to release the food nutrients properly.

8 EAT AT THE TABLE

Sit at the table when it's time to eat. I want you to focus on what you are eating and sitting on the sofa in front of the TV is about as mindless as it can get. At the table, you will eat more slowly, feel more full; and sitting up straight helps digestion. Don't be a mindless muncher!

9 KEEP MOVING

Walking to the shops, mowing the lawn and taking the stairs
at work all count and keep you moving throughout the day.
See pages 74–84 for my exercise programme and also remember
the more you move, the more pounds you will lose.

10 DON'T SHOP WHEN YOU'RE HUNGRY

You'll end up buying all kinds of things you know you shouldn't.
Eat something before you go, make a shopping list and stick to it.

11 BE PREPARED

Be prepared in order to avoid temptation. Take healthy lunches
and snacks to work such as fruit, vegetable sticks and dips,
soups, salads, bean sprouts, nuts, seeds, rye bread, oat cakes,
avocados, nut butters, leftovers from dinner and herbal tea bags.

12 EAT IN THE RAW

Every time you have something cooked, have something raw
with it. Even if you make soup, you must add raw herbs or veg
at the end. Raw foods are the only source of food enzymes,
a catalyst for weight balance.

13 BLEND THE DAY AWAY

Eat lots of blended soups, e.g. sweet potato and squash. These
are easy to digest. Fruit smoothies are great too. Make them
for breakfast.

14 SUPPLEMENTS

Weight Loss Helper Guide:

VITAMIN B COMPLEX Essential for efficient metabolism of carbs and proteins. 50mg daily.

ASTRAGALUS Packed with Vitamin B, it enhances adrenal function which is critical for weight loss. Get it in tincture form, put into hot water and drink. 15 drops twice daily for 3 months.

SIBERIAN GINSENG Helps to stabilize blood sugar and diminish cravings. 15 drops twice daily for 3 months.

CO-ENZYME Q10 Helps stimulate the metabolism and weight loss. 150mg daily.

DIGESTIVE ENZYME SUPPLEMENTS: Help boost nutrient uptake and suppress appetite. One with lunch and one with dinner.

RAW SHELLED HEMP SEEDS AND OIL Provides exactly the right combination of essential fatty acids to boost metabolism and weight loss. 1 or 2 tablespoons of seeds daily or every other day. 1 tablespoon of oil drizzled over a raw salad.

KELP Helps support the thyroid gland and aid weight loss. Follow directions on the label.

ALOE VERA JUICE Has a soothing effect on the stomach. Take before meals and follow instructions on the label.

DR GILLIAN MCKEITH'S LIVING FOOD ENERGY POWDER Packed full of vitamins, enzymes, minerals, antioxidants, amino acids, essential fatty acids and co-factors. 1 or 2 teaspoons a day added to water or fruit juice.

LECITHIN GRANULES Helps utilize body fat. You can sprinkle them over salads. 2 teaspoons once a week.

CHICKWEED Helps break down fat deposits that are hard to shift. 15–30 drops of the tincture or 500mg capsule daily (take before meals).

NETTLE TEA A great weight loss tea as it boosts metabolism and is a natural appetite suppressant. Alternate with dandelion tea and drink 3–4 cups daily.

RED RASPBERRY LEAF TEA May help to reduce appetite and tastes good.

SPIRULINA Rich in protein, this can help control blood sugar swings and food cravings. 6 tablets daily or 1 teaspoon of the powder form mixed in juice.

NOTE: ALWAYS CONSULT WITH YOUR GP BEFORE TAKING SUPPLEMENTS.

15 BREAKFAST LIKE A KING

Eat breakfast like a king, lunch like a queen and dinner like
a pauper. Make sure you eat more at lunchtime than for dinner.

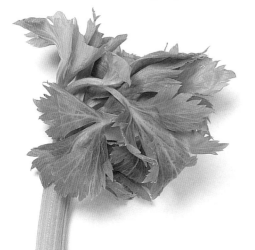

16 EARLY TO BED

Get to bed by 10:30pm. Your liver and gallbladder need to do
their detoxing work between 11pm and 2pm. Healthy livers help
balance weight. Studies show that sleeping before midnight and
having regular sleeping and waking times is healthiest for the
body. You need a good eight hours sleep. Being tired slows your
metabolism and can affect your food choices, making you go for
high calorie, fatty foods for a fast, brief, energy burst.

17 EAT AT REGULAR TIMES

Try to eat breakfast, lunch, dinner and snacks around the
same time each day. Irregular eating habits can cause bloating.
If you leave your stomach empty for long periods of time the
secretion of digestive enzymes slows down. Irregular eating
habits can also play havoc with your blood sugar and you need
a stable blood sugar level to keep you from gaining weight.

18 EAT DINNER EARLY

Dinner should be no later than 6 to 7pm, if possible. Unless you want to gain weight and feel sluggish, of course.

19 EAT WHEN CALM

If you are upset, wait until the feeling passes or lessens and then eat. Do not attempt to eat a full meal if you are stressed out or upset. Best to opt for vegetable juices or simple soups that day as they are much easier on the digestion.

20 THROW OUT YOUR SCALES

In all the years that I have been working with people who want to lose weight, I have never weighed anybody. People are too obsessed with weight. I don't do the weight thing. Instead, I put you on a whole new lifestyle. I never weigh a person and nor do I get them calorie counting or portion controlling. You don't need to be a biophysicist or a mathematician to embark upon my journey.

If you want to have a positive, passionate relationship with food, you have to look at food in a whole different way. My Plan will allow your body to find its natural weight. But depriving yourself and saving up calories for unhealthy foods is a recipe for disaster. Give up the weighing and counting and release yourself.

THE SMOOTHIE SEMINAR

I consider myself the Queen of Smoothies. It's my number
one choice for breakfast. My best friends make fun of me because
my blender works overtime. If you come into my kitchen, you hear
constant whirring as I blend and blend. In meetings, I often have
a smoothie, on trains I always have containers of smoothies.
I absolutely love to make them because they are so easy to toss
together, they fill you up, are a cinch to digest and taste delicious.

Smoothies are the perfect introduction to healthy eating.
Low-cal, low fat and high energy, they make a wonderful breakfast,
light meal or snack. So to give yourself a really easy way in to the
Dr Gillian lifestyle, think smoothies and get your blenders to
the ready!

Good smoothies are generally thick and full-bodied. I like mine
to have a pudding consistency, almost like yoghurt. Juicers extract
only the juice from fruit and leave the pulp behind – with a smoothie
you use a blender and nothing goes to waste. They are so easy to
prepare and so good for you. For example, throw into a blender a ripe
peach or nectarine, a banana and some strawberries, then blend
for a minute or so, and voilà! you've got the hang of it. You are done!

Just be creative. The key is to experiment and have fun with it.
And if you prefer to make your smoothie thinner, just add extra
water or a watery fruit. You could even try adding a grain milk
for an all-natural super smoothie milkshake. Or add a sprinkle
of cinnamon for extra taste. Whatever you fancy.

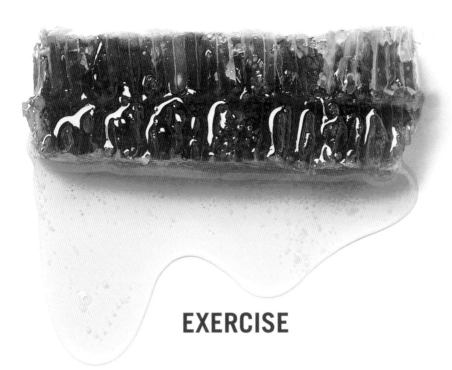

EXERCISE

Have you ever noticed, when you are greeted by someone their first sentence is often, 'Take a seat?' Why are we so obsessed with sitting? Every single person I have ever met who wants to lose weight does not move nearly enough. They get inside their cars and sit. They go to work and sit at a desk, then they go home and sit again. Our bodies are not designed to sit on sofas, slump at desks, slob out in front of the television, or stare at a computer screen hour after hour without moving. We need to transform ourselves from a nation of sitters to a nation of movers and shakers. The acceptance of a sedentary life is downright wrong and we must change it.

Exercise is something that needs to be done continuously, all the time, every day. It's not enough to just fit it in once or twice a week, although even that's preferable to no exercise at all. I want you to move your body as much as you possibly can, throughout the day. This part of my lifestyle is non-negotiable. I am not asking you to become a fitness fanatic, but if you want to be slim and healthy then you need a positive attitude to exercise. I won't hear any excuses. There is no getting around me on this!

Break the Vicious Cycle

Lack of exercise is one of the most serious health issues facing the Western world today. And lack of movement is a vicious cycle. The less you move, the less you want to move, the less you are ultimately able to move.

When you eat the new Dr Gillian way, you are introducing many more nutrients, vitamins, minerals, amino acids, proteins, phytonutrients and essential fatty acids into your body and cells. The only truly effective way to properly distribute all of these new nutrients throughout your system is via exercise. Exercising before meals increases metabolism and enables you to burn your food more effectively. Once you start this good habit, you will not want to stop it.

Your new lifestyle should include an attitude to exercise which is constant – you should always be looking to keep active: cycle to the shops, walk to the supermarket, take the stairs, jog to the cinema, dance to music every night, stretch and skip rope outside, buy a hula hoop and learn to use it, bounce on a trampoline.

On the Plan you need to incorporate some form of exercise into every day. I'm not expecting you to be a fitness fanatic, but even 30 minutes a day of moderate activity will reap huge rewards. Regular exercise:

▸ **Gets your circulation going and makes you feel alive**
▸ **Speeds up metabolism and helps burn fat**
▸ **Releases endorphins which improve mood**
▸ **Increases your energy levels and improves sleep patterns**
▸ **Improves overall fitness and your ability to fight off colds and minor ailments**
▸ **Makes you feel good about yourself**

YOUR EXERCISE COMMITMENT

I require three exercise commitments from you. Place your signature in the box provided under each statement. This is your promise to me and to yourself.

One:

I agree to move my body every day through exercise.
Signature ....

Some days you may move and exercise more than other days. The important thing is that you do move.

Two:

I agree to exercise before each meal.

Signature ....

This can be as simple as brisk walking. You walk for 20 minutes before breakfast, 20 minutes before lunch and walk or dance for 20 minutes before dinner. Or you might run in place or jump up and down on a mini trampoline for 10 minutes before your meal. (You may need to work up gradually to a full 20-minute walk or 10-minute run or trampoline.)

Three:

I agree to use a mini trampoline, swim or join and use a gym regularly.

Signature ....

This is your insurance policy against bad weather. I don't want to hear that it was raining and you could not walk anywhere. If you are seriously overweight, you may have to lose a certain amount before you can get on a mini trampoline. In the meantime, try swimming. The water supports your body and takes all the stress off your joints while you concentrate on working those muscles. Joining a gym can be a fantastic motivator and a good way to meet like-minded people. Of course, you have to actually go to the gym and use it. Maybe two or three days a week you are at the gym, and you do some other exercise on the other days.

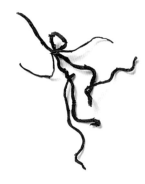

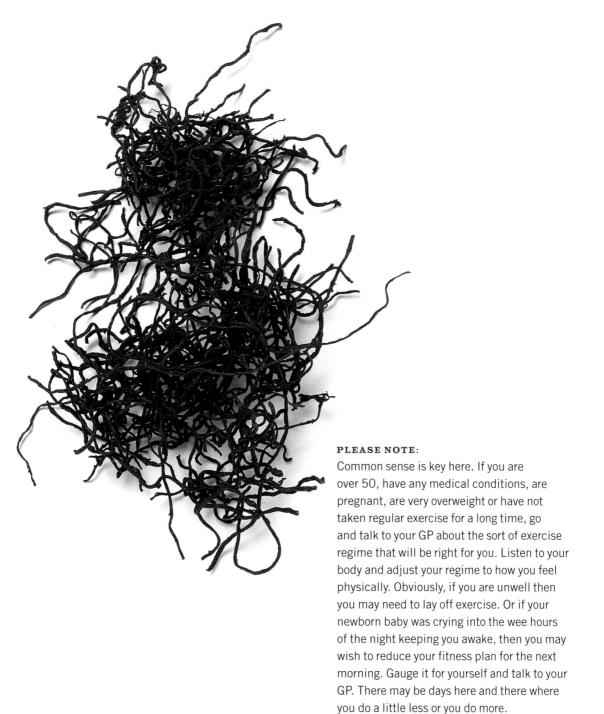

PLEASE NOTE:
Common sense is key here. If you are
over 50, have any medical conditions, are
pregnant, are very overweight or have not
taken regular exercise for a long time, go
and talk to your GP about the sort of exercise
regime that will be right for you. Listen to your
body and adjust your regime to how you feel
physically. Obviously, if you are unwell then
you may need to lay off exercise. Or if your
newborn baby was crying into the wee hours
of the night keeping you awake, then you may
wish to reduce your fitness plan for the next
morning. Gauge it for yourself and talk to your
GP. There may be days here and there where
you do a little less or you do more.

Do It Daily

You need to do something every day, no matter how small. Depending on your starting weight and stamina, do one minute, work up to five minutes, 10 minutes, 15 minutes. Gradually and slowly work up to at least 30 minutes and then up to an hour, four to six times a week. But you would still move on the seventh day. Some days you can do more or less exercise than others. So maybe five days a week you are doing some form of exercise for up to an hour a day, and on the other two days you are doing only 20 minutes. Are you catching my point here? I want you to adapt the exercise to your abilities and also how you are feeling on that particular day. Our bodies are very dynamic organisms and we need to adjust to that dynamism. The old adage, 'No pain, no gain,' does not apply here. My exercise programme is not about hurting or killing your body. I want your exercise to be in harmony and in tune with your muscles, endurance levels and frame.

Often, when they hear me give a seminar, people get excited about an exercise programme. After 20 years of not moving, they want to jog for miles straight off. This could be a great way to do yourself in. This type of person might be incapacitated for weeks because they have weakened their body and stressed their muscles. The aches and pains will be harrowing. This is not what I want.

Stick With It

Getting to 30 minutes of exercise and eventually up to an hour or more five, six or seven times a week may take several weeks or even a few months to achieve. Just stick with it and you'll soon find that your fitness levels and your enjoyment increase. If you don't think you can find a spare 30 minutes or so at one time, try to include several short bouts of activity in a day, say three 10-minute sessions at first, working up to three 20-minute sessions. You are then exercising for an hour a day. Exercise must be:

- **Consistent**
- **Performed every single day in some form**
- **Varied**
- **Adapted to how you feel that day**

WHAT KIND OF EXERCISE?

A combination of aerobic exercise and resistance/flexibility training is ideal:

- **Aerobic – walking, jogging, swimming, cycling, rowing, dancing, skating, trampolining**
- **Resistance and flexibility – yoga, Pilates, weights, resistance exercises (e.g. press ups)**

My best advice is to vary the exercise for two reasons:
1. It is better for the muscles and the body.
2. It prevents boredom and keeps you more interested.

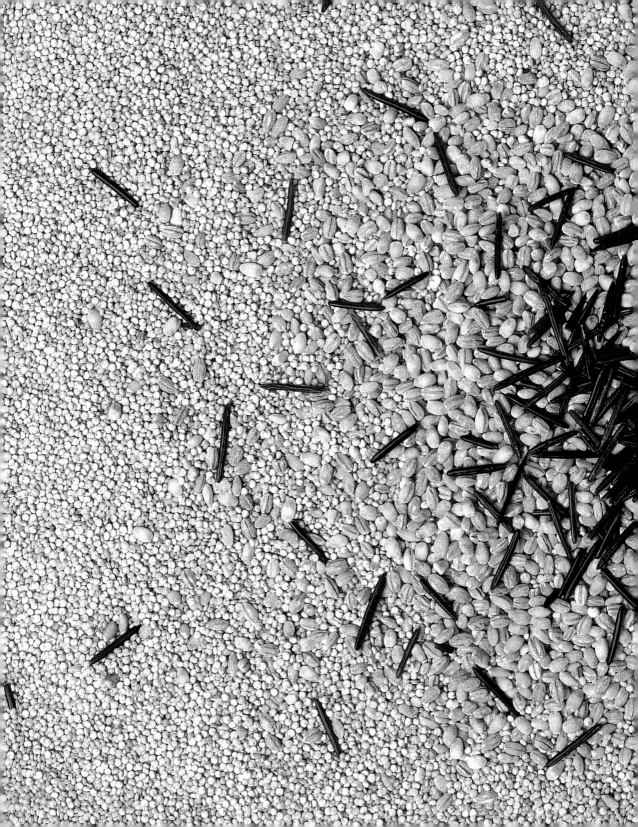

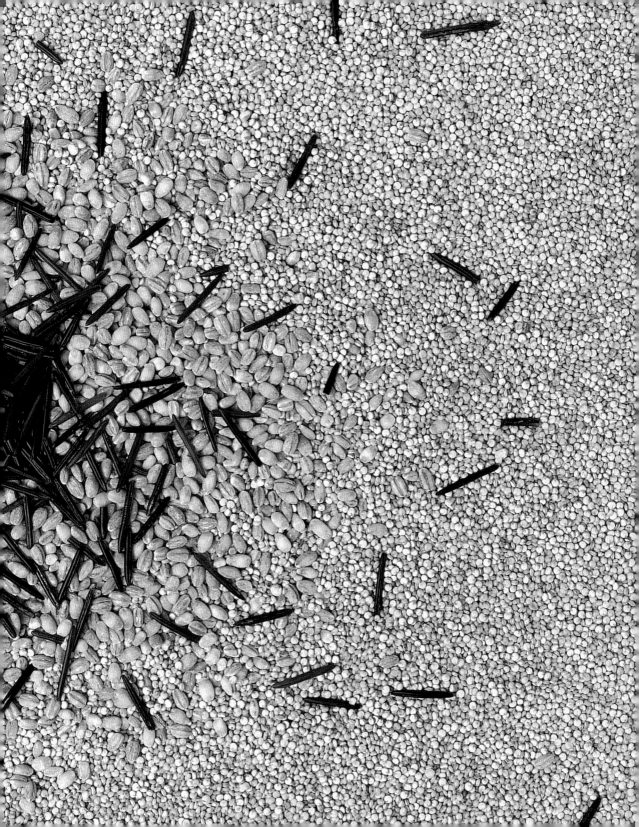

EXERCISE PLAN FOR BEGINNERS

Walking

Walking is one of my favourite forms of exercise. No expertise or equipment is required. You can do it anytime and it's free! Provided you do it regularly and for long enough, walking can be just as beneficial as any of the more vigorous activities (like jogging or trampolining).

HOW TO START

Take a 10-minute walk, twice a day.

- ► Gradually extend yourself:
- ► Walk every day
- ► Walk longer
- ► Walk faster
- ► Walk and swing your arms at the same time
- ► Walk up one or two gentle slopes
- ► Walk up steeper slopes

Ideally I would like you to work up to walking for one hour. You can break that hour up into three sets of 20 minutes, 20 minutes before breakfast, 20 minutes before lunch and 20 minutes before dinner.

Swimming

For most people, especially those who are very overweight, swimming is even better than walking. Similar to walking, start by going to the pool twice a week for a gentle 15-minute swim. When I swim, I count the number of lengths of the pool I swim. Start with one length of the pool and comfortably and gradually increase the number of lengths and your work rate while in the water. Aim to build up to about 30 minutes a day, or 45 minutes twice or three times a week.

Cycling, Trampolining, Going to the Gym or Jogging

Your aim is the same as for walking or swimming. Start with a short easy routine – 10 to 15 minutes per day and slowly work up to about 30 minutes a day. Gradually increase your work rate without ever straining yourself.

Apart from the fact that jumping up and down makes you feel like a kid again, trampolining causes every cell in the body to respond. Balance, reflexes and circulation improve, your colon is stimulated, body toned, muscles strengthened and feet massaged.

When I go to the gym I sometimes see people spending untold minutes and hours on the one machine. If you go to the gym, then vary the exercises. For example, do 10 minutes of the walking machine, 10 minutes of the stairs, 10 minutes of lifting weights and so on. This way, you vary your workout, don't get bored and get all the benefits.

If jogging, please invest in a good pair of running shoes that offer cushioned support and, if you're a woman, for all activities invest in a good sports bra.

Is there anything I should do before and after I exercise?

► Make sure that you drink adequate fluids in advance of your exercise otherwise you run the risk of becoming dehydrated and ending up with a headache.

► Start an exercise session with a gradual warm-up period. During this time (about 5 to 10 minutes), you should slowly stretch your muscles first and then gradually increase your level of activity. For example, begin walking slowly and then pick up the pace.

► After you are finished exercising, cool down for about 5 to 10 minutes. If you have been jogging, slow down to a gentle walk before stopping. You are stretching your muscles and allowing your heart rate to slow down gradually. You can use the same stretches as in the warm-up period.

HOW HARD DO I HAVE TO EXERCISE?

Even small amounts of exercise are better than none at all.
Start with an activity you can do comfortably. As a rule of thumb
when you are exercising you should be slightly out of breath
but not so out of breath that you can't hold a conversation with
someone. So if you find yourself panting, huffing and puffing
within a few minutes, stop. You're exercising too hard.

HOW DO I STAY MOTIVATED?

FIND A FITNESS PARTNER Find a walking
partner, play tennis with your spouse or
a friend, or go rollerblading with the kids.

SCHEDULE YOUR WORKOUTS Exercise
must be a priority in order to establish
it as a lifestyle practice. Make time
for your workouts and schedule them
on your daily calendar or planner.

DRESS THE PART Wear comfortable
clothes appropriate for exercising.
They will help you feel like working
out. If you exercise at a gym, put your
exercise wear in a bag and set it beside
the door the night before. When it's
time to head out the door, all you have
to do is grab your bag on the way out.

ENTERTAIN YOURSELF If you exercise
alone, consider using a portable music
device to listen to your favourite music
or books on tape to help keep you
entertained during your workout. Many
pieces of exercise equipment have racks
that fit onto the console to hold reading
material. If you exercise at home, turn
on some music or bring the television
within viewing range.

MAKE EXERCISE NON-NEGOTIABLE
Think of exercise as something you
do without question, like brushing
your teeth or going to work. Taking
this lifestyle perspective will help
you make exercise a habit.
WARNING! NEVER OVERDO EXERCISE!

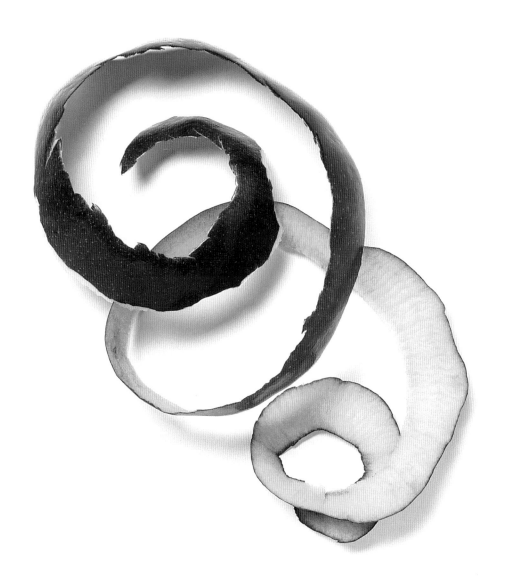

DR GILLIAN'S FAT FLUSH

FAT FLUSH FOR WEIGHT LOSS

If you are overweight, you could get your plan started with my two-day detox followed by the Fat Flush day. This will help cleanse your system and make the 28-day plan even more effective.

BREAKFAST

A cup of warm water with a squeeze of lemon and lime
Two whole pink grapefruit

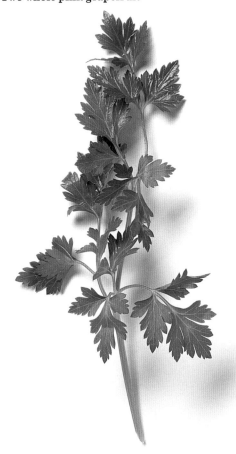

LUNCH
Mung Bean Casserole with Special Brown Rice

Mung Bean Casserole
SERVES 2
125g mung beans
500ml water or vegetable stock
plus water to soak
1 tsp fennel seeds
1 onion, finely chopped
2 carrots, peeled and diced
2 tbsp flat leaf parsley, chopped
1 endive
handful clover sprouts

1. Soak the mung beans in 1 litre of cold water for 6 hours. Drain and rinse well. Bring the water or stock to the boil, add the beans and simmer for 10 minutes. Skim away any white scum that rises to the surface.
2. Add the fennel seeds and simmer for 10 minutes. Then add the onion and carrots and simmer for a further 10 minutes.
3. Remove from the heat and add the parsley.
4. Arrange the endive leaves around the edge of two soup bowls, pour the casserole in the centre of the bowls, sprinkle over the clover sprouts and serve with Special Brown Rice.

Special Brown Rice
100g brown rice
1 onion, peeled and chopped
200ml water
1/2 tsp turmeric
1/2 tsp cumin

1. Place the rice, spices and onion in a saucepan. Add 200ml water.
2. Bring the water to the boil, lower heat and simmer for 20 minutes.
3. Turn off the heat and allow to stand for 10 minutes before serving.

DINNER
Chilled Cucumber Soup with Coleslaw Salad

Chilled Cucumber Soup
SERVES 2
3 cucumbers
4 spring onions, finely sliced
500ml water
juice of half a lemon
6-8 mint leaves
50g sprouting beans

1. Cut one cucumber in half and finely dice, reserve for the garnish.
2. Take the remaining cucumbers, peel, halve and with a teaspoon remove the seeds and discard.
3. Place the deseeded cucumbers in a food processor with the spring onions and water, and blend until smooth.
4. Add the lemon juice and mint leaves and blend again.
5. Pout into bowls and chill well. Serve with sprouting beans and diced cucumber sprinkled over the top.

Coleslaw Salad
1 carrot trimmed
1 spring onion
10g walnut pieces
small piece of white cabbage, cored and shredded
1 celery stalk
1 tbsp chopped coriander or chopped parsley
15g fresh garden peas
3 radishes, finely chopped
FOR THE DRESSING, BLEND THE FOLLOWING:
4 tbsp hemp oil
1 handful rocket leaves
2 tbsp pine nuts
1 garlic clove, peeled and crushed

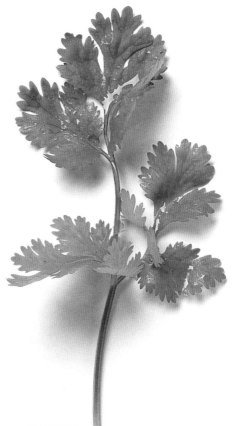

EVENING
Mix 200ml of pink grapefruit juice and 2 tbsp of olive oil or hemp oil and drink.

Drink warm cups of water throughout the day. Alternate between sage tea and a herbal tea called Pau D'arco tea during the day (available from health food stores).

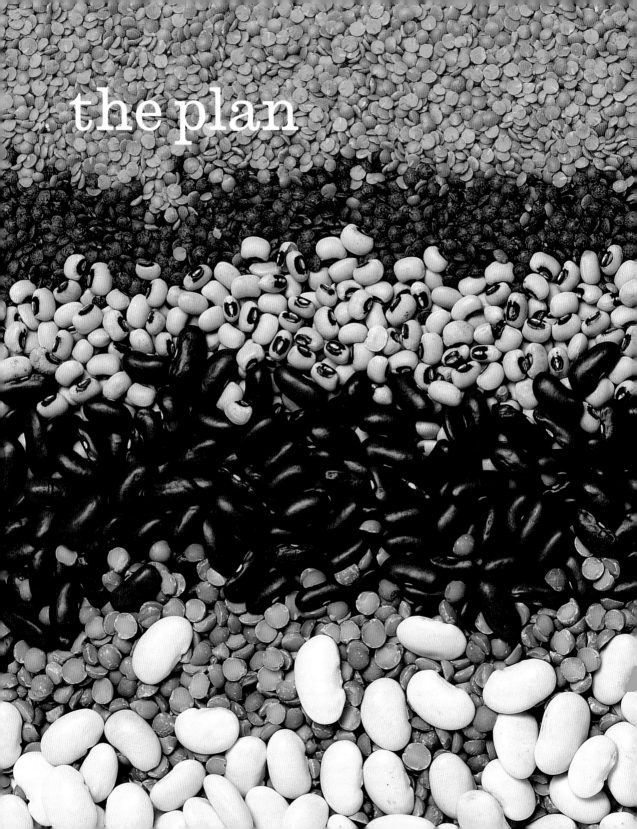

the plan

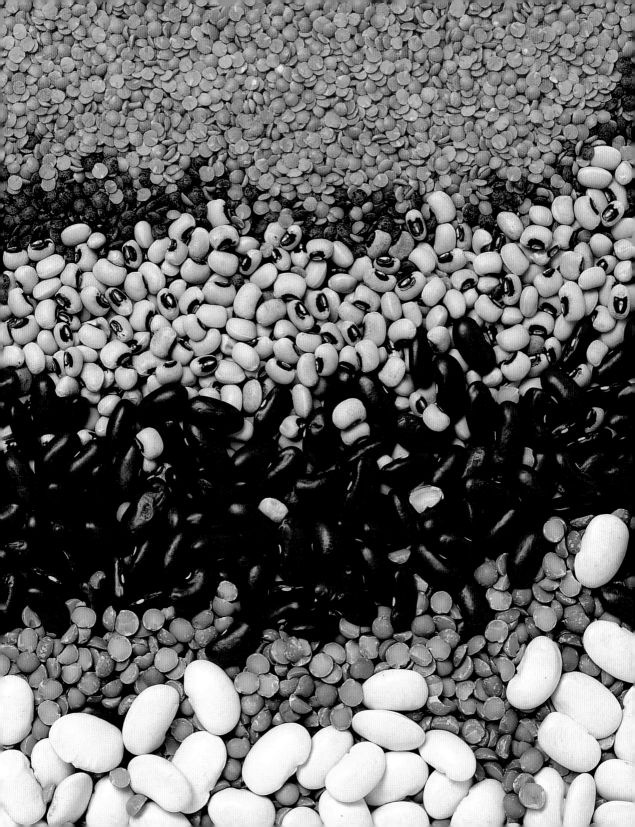

Day 1

BREAKFAST

1 cup of warm water with a squeeze of lemon
1 cup Nettle tea
followed by fruit salad and a bowl
of Easy Oats.

Fruit Berry Salad
SERVES 1
1 small tub blueberries
1 small tub raspberries
1 small punnet strawberries

Easy Oats
If you are still hungry, you can have
a bowl of porridge oats, but you need to
wait 20 minutes to let your fruit digest.

SERVES 1
100g porridge oats
400ml water or rice milk

1. Combine the porridge oats with
the water or rice milk in a pan.
2. Bring to the boil, then lower the heat
and simmer for 15–20 minutes.
3. Season with a sprinkle of cinnamon.

MID-MORNING SNACK
Veggie Juice or two celery stalks with dip
(see page 200 for dips).

Veggie Juice
SERVES 1
2 celery stalks
6 carrots

LUNCH

Tuna and Leafy Salad
SERVES 1
1 small bag watercress,
spinach and rocket leaf salad
200-g can tuna steak in spring water
handful of halved cherry tomatoes
a few slices cucumber
1–2 tbsp chopped, fresh dill
squeeze of lemon juice

1. Shake the bag of leaf salad into a bowl.
2. Top with the drained can of tuna steak.
Flake into chunks with a fork.
3. Add the halved cherry tomatoes,
cucumber and dill.
4. Drizzle with freshly squeezed lemon
juice before serving.

MID-AFTERNOON SNACK
Veggie Juice or one whole yellow pepper, finely chopped.

Veggie Juice
SERVES 1
6 celery stalks
1 cucumber
1 yellow pepper

DINNER

Poached Chicken in Ginger Miso with Bok Choy

SERVES 1

1 free range chicken breast
300ml vegetable stock or make
stock with a veggie cube
1 tbsp organic miso
1–2cm piece of fresh ginger
2 cloves garlic, peeled and chopped
3 tbsps fresh coriander
½ red pepper, finely sliced
1 handful beansprouts
2 Bok Choy trimmed and roughly
chopped, save 2 leaves for garnish

1. Preheat oven to 200C/Gas Mark 6. Take a large sheet of foil and place the chicken in the centre.
2. In a small pan, bring the stock to the boil and add the miso, ginger, garlic and 1 tbsp of the coriander.
3. Pull the foil up to create a bowl shape and spoon over the flavoured stock. Scrunch the foil up to create a parcel. Transfer to a baking tray and cook for 10 minutes.
4. Arrange the Bok Choy on a serving plate. Transfer the cooked chicken on to the Bok Choy and then sprinkle over the pepper and sprouts.
5. Garnish with the two whole leaves of Bok Choy and remaining coriander. Serve immediately.

VEGETARIAN ALTERNATIVE
Marinated Veggie Tofu

SERVES 2

175g chilled tofu, cut into 1.5cm cubes
1 medium carrot, sliced
1 red pepper, sliced
75g sugar-snap peas
60g broccoli florets
20g cashew nuts
2 spring onions, finely sliced

FOR THE MARINADE

2 tbsps wheat-free Tamari sauce
1 garlic clove, peeled and crushed
1 tsp finely chopped fresh root ginger

1. Mix the marinade in a shallow dish and marinate the tofu for 10 minutes.
2. Stir-fry the carrot, pepper, sugar-snap peas, and broccoli with cold pressed sunflower oil and a little water, for 3 minutes.
3. Lift the tofu out of the marinade with a slotted spoon and add to the pan with the cashew nuts and spring onions.
4. Stir-fry for 1–2 minutes, turning gently until the tofu is hot.

Drink a cup of warm water an hour before bed every day of the Plan.

Day 2

1 cup of warm water
1 cup Dandelion tea
followed by a smoothie.

Peach and Mango Smoothie
SERVES 1
1 large mango, stoned and chopped
1 peach, stoned and chopped
1 banana, sliced
200ml water
1 small tub blueberries

1. Blend all ingredients
(except blueberries) until smooth.
2. Add more water if you want
a thinner consistency.
3. Pour over the blueberries and drink.

MID-MORNING SNACK
Bowl of grapes.

LUNCH
Miso Soup followed by Avocado and Pine Nut Salad.

Miso Soup
Simply add miso powder to a mug of water
and drink. There are different flavours of
miso, and some miso packs come with tofu
added too. So easy.

Avocado and Pine Nut Salad
SERVES 2
2 little gem lettuces
1 avocado
4 tomatoes, quartered
1 red pepper, sliced
1 yellow pepper, sliced
handful of fresh basil leaves
handful of alfalfa sprouts (optional)
handful of radishes (optional)
2 tbsp extra virgin olive oil or hemp oil
3 tbsp pine nuts

1. Separate and wash the lettuce leaves.
2. Place the lettuce in a large bowl with the
avocado, tomatoes, peppers, and basil leaves.
3. If possible add a generous serving of
alfalfa sprouts and decorate with a handful
of radishes.
4. Drizzle with 2 tbsp of extra virgin olive
oil or hemp oil and sprinkle with 2–3 tbsp
pine nuts.

MID-AFTERNOON SNACK
Cucumber and carrot crudités with houmous,
sprinkled with dill.

Keep smelling sweet from your insides with a mango. Mango acts like an internal deodorant because it contains antioxidants that can help eliminate odour-causing bacteria.

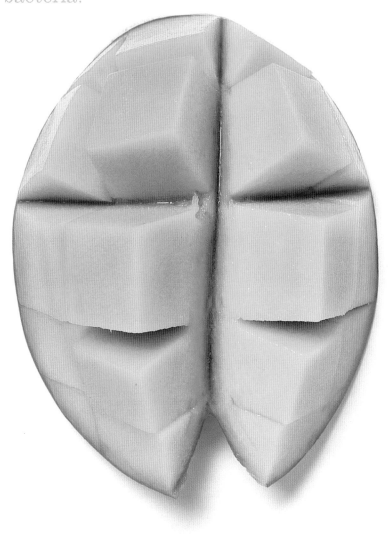

Poached Monkfish with Tarragon

You can use any firm, white fish, but monkfish is particularly good. With all the recipes, don't fret if you can't find a particular ingredient, I just want to give you lots of ideas.

SERVES 2
140g baby spinach leaves
2 vine ripened tomatoes, sliced
500ml water
1 bay leaf
1-2cm piece fresh ginger, peeled
1 lemon grass stalk
2 cloves garlic, peeled
1 Kaffir lime leaf, or juice of lime
1 tsp fresh miso paste
200g piece fresh monkfish
large handful fresh tarragon
1 dsp olive oil

1. Arrange the baby spinach and tomatoes on a serving plate.
2. Bring the water to the boil with the bay leaf, ginger, lemon grass, garlic, Kaffir lime leaf and miso paste. Boil for 5 minutes and then reduce to a simmer.
3. Poach the fish for 3–4 minutes or until firm to the touch.
4. Remove the fish from the pan and keep it warm while you finish the sauce.
5. Boil the liquid until the volume has reduced by half.
6. Remove from the heat and strain in a small bowl, discarding the seasoning.
7. Add the tarragon and oil, and with a hand-held blender blitz until smooth. Alternatively this can be done in a small processor.
8. Place the fish on the spinach and tomatoes, spoon over the sauce and serve.

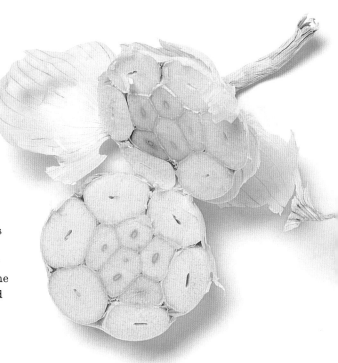

Day 3

BREAKFAST

1 cup of warm water with a squeeze of lemon
1 cup Nettle tea
followed by a smoothie.

Strawberry Smoothie
SERVES 1
1 small punnet strawberries, hulled
1/2 small tub raspberries
2 ripe pears, cored and chopped
1 apple, peeled and chopped
200ml water

Blend all the ingredients until smooth.

MID-MORNING SNACK
Four chicory leaves, topped with houmous and baby tomatoes.

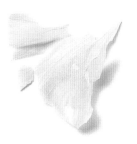

LUNCH
Baked Sweet Potato with sprouted alfalfa seeds and a Beetroot Salad.

Sweet Potato
Pop a large sweet potato into the oven for 30 minutes while you prepare your salad.

Beetroot Salad
Baby beetroot are best for this salad but you can use larger beetroot and peel them before making the salad.

SERVES 1
500g baby beetroot
1 tbsp cider vinegar
1/2 cucumber, finely sliced
1 tbsp sesame seeds
2 tbsp alfalfa sprouts

1. Scrub the beetroot well and trim the stalks to about 3–4 cm in length and then place in a steamer and cook for 7–10 minutes. The time will depend on the size of the beetroot.
2. Allow the beetroot to cool slightly then cut in half and arrange on a serving plate with the cucumber.
3. Pour over the vinegar, sprinkle with the sesame seeds and alfalfa sprouts, and serve.

MID-AFTERNOON SNACK
Veggie Juice or a handful of salt-free organic almonds (if you can soak the almonds first in water they will be even easier to digest).

Veggie Juice
SERVES 1
4 carrots
1/2 beetroot
2 celery stalks

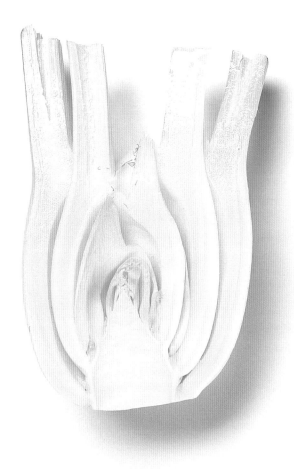

Soup with Lemon and Fennel Coleslaw.

White Bean Soup

My creamy white bean soup is perfect if you miss soups with cream in them. Coriander seeds are available in health food shops and can be ground in a clean pepper grinder. Reserve a portion for lunch tomorrow.

SERVES 4
1 onion, peeled and chopped
2 leeks, sliced
2 cloves garlic, peeled and chopped
1 tsp olive oil
500ml vegetable stock or water
2 bay leaves
small bunch parsley stalks
freshly ground coriander seeds
450-g can cannelini beans, drained
fresh chives to garnish

1. Place the onion, leeks, garlic, oil and a little water in a medium sized pan. Cook over a moderate heat for 5 minutes until the vegetables are slightly softened. Do not allow the vegetables to colour.
2. Bring the vegetable stock to the boil and pour over the vegetables. Add the bay leaves and parsley. Season with the coriander seeds.
3. Return the soup to the boil and simmer for 15 minutes.
4. Add the beans for 3–4 minutes on a very low heat until they are warmed through.
5. Remove the pan from the heat and allow to cool slightly. Remove the bay leaf then blend with a stick blender or in the food processor.
6. Spoon into warmed deep soup bowls. Sprinkle with fresh chives and serve immediately.

Lemon and Fennel Coleslaw

SERVES 2
350g red cabbage
1 fennel bulb, trimmed and finely sliced
2 celery sticks, trimmed and sliced
2 spring onions, trimmed and sliced
4 tbsp freshly squeezed lemon juice
3 tbsp extra virgin olive oil
50g walnut halves, roughly chopped

1. Remove the outer leaves of the cabbage
and cut out and discard the central core.
2. Slice the cabbage very finely and place
in a serving bowl – you should have around
275g prepared weight.
3. Add the fennel, celery, spring onions,
lemon juice and oil. Toss well together and
sprinkle with the walnuts just before serving.

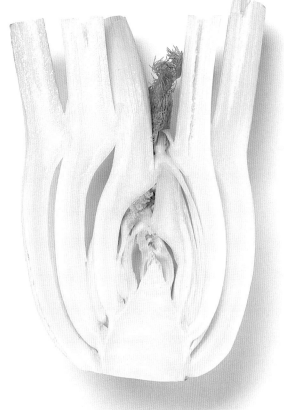

Fennel removes fat and
mucus from the intestinal
tract and acts like a natural
appetite suppressant.

Day 4

BREAKFAST

1 cup of warm water
1 cup **Dandelion tea**
followed by fruit salad and Savoury Quinoa.

Fruit Salad
1 apple
1 pear
1 peach
2 apricots

Savoury Quinoa
Use the grain, not the flakes. Remember
to allow 20 minutes between eating your
fruit and your porridge. If you are in a rush,
pour the quinoa into a container and take
it to work.

SERVES 1–2
150g quinoa
350ml water
2 tsp sesame seeds
dried mixed herbs (optional)

1. Put the quinoa and water in a pan.
Bring to boil and simmer for 8 minutes.
2. Allow the porridge to sit for a few
minutes and serve.
3. Garnish with dried mixed herbs if you
need extra flavour.

MID-MORNING SNACK
Juice of two whole pink grapefruit.

LUNCH
White Bean Soup from the night before, with Zesty
Avocado Mayo served with vegetable crudités (raw veggies
chopped in strips or bite-size chunks for dipping).

Zesty Avocado Mayo
It keeps well in the fridge for 24 hours.

SERVES 2
1 ripe avocado
$^{1}/_{2}$ tsp finely grated lemon zest
2 tbsp freshly squeezed lemon juice

1. Blend all the ingredients together using
a stick blender until smooth and creamy
(or mash very well with a fork). Add a little
more lemon juice if liked.
2. Spoon into a small dish and cover the
surface tightly with non-PVC cling film
to prevent browning.
3. Chill until ready to serve.

MID-AFTERNOON SNACK
Bowl of cherries.

DINNER

Adzuki Bean Bake with Savoy cabbage, green beans or broccoli.

It's that time again. Ah yes. It's time for the Adzuki beans! You cannot escape Adzuki beans à la Dr Gillian! But this new recipe is a whole new way to get these healthy beans into you.

Adzuki Bean Bake

This recipe makes two generous servings, so save some for the next day's lunch.

SERVES 2

1 tbsp olive oil, plus extra for brushing
1 medium onion, peeled and chopped
2 garlic cloves, peeled and crushed
1 small squash, peeled and diced
1 large carrot, peeled and diced
1 celery stick, trimmed and sliced
500ml just-boiled water
1 tsp organic vegetable bouillon (stock) powder
165g cooked adzuki beans
1 medium leek, trimmed and sliced
2 tsp cornflour or arrowroot blended with 1 tbsp cold water to make a smooth paste
1 large sweet potato, cut into 5mm slices. (If you like a lot of topping, use 2 potatoes)

1. Heat the oil in a large saucepan with a tiny bit of water, so you are water sautéing really. You are not frying in the normal sense of the word.
2. Gently water sauté the onion and garlic for 3 minutes, stirring occasionally.
3. Add the squash, carrot and celery. Cook with the onion and garlic for 2 minutes, stirring regularly.
4. Pour the just-boiled water over the vegetables and stir in the bouillon powder.
5. Bring to the boil, then reduce the heat and simmer for 10 minutes.
6. Preheat the oven to 200C/Gas 6.
7. Stir the sliced leek and adzuki beans into the vegetable mixture. Return to a simmer and cook for 5 minutes, stirring occasionally.
8. Add the cornflour or arrowroot mixture and cook for about 1 minute until the sauce thickens, stirring.
9. Remove from the heat and transfer carefully into a 900ml ovenproof dish.
10. Arrange slices of the sweet potato on top of the bean and vegetable mixture. Brush with a little of the oil and bake for about 30 minutes until the potato is soft.
11. Serve with freshly cooked Savoy cabbage, green beans or broccoli and raw mangetout.

Hail to the Adzuki Bean, my Bean of Weight Loss. Packed with weight-regulating nutrients, Adzuki beans act like a sponge soaking up excess fluid in the body. Adzukis are my bean of choice for you for weight loss. Eat them at least once a week.

Day 5

BREAKFAST

1 cup of warm water with a squeeze of lemon
1 cup Slippery Elm tea
followed by vegetable juice.

Ginger Zinger
If you are running late, pour the juice into
a container with a straw and drink it on
the way.

SERVES 1
6 carrots
1/2 tsp chopped ginger
1 cucumber
1 stick of celery

1. Push all the ingredients through the
hopper of the juicer and pour into a glass.
2. Sip slowly.

REMEMBER TO LEAVE YOUR YELLOW SPLIT PEAS TO
SOAK IN PLENTY OF WATER READY FOR THE EVENING.

MID-MORNING SNACK
Two peaches.

LUNCH
Adzuki Bean Bake from last night, heat and serve on a bed
of raw leaves, herbs and sprouted seeds of your choice.

MID-AFTERNOON SNACK
Veggie Juice or one fennel bulb, chopped and served
with a dip (see page 200 for dips).

Veggie Juice
SERVES 1
1 fennel
1/2 beetroot
1 cucumber

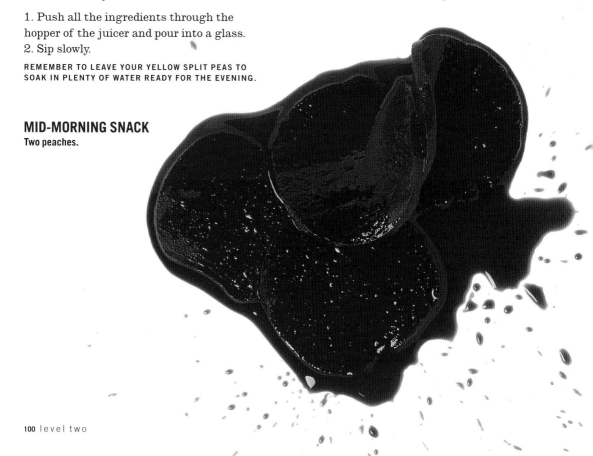

DINNER
Soup and Chinese Style Salad.

Easy Peasy Yellow Pea Soup
Save a portion for lunch tomorrow.

SERVES 4
225g yellow split peas, soaked for 3 hours
1 sweet potato
2 carrots
2 onions
1 tbsp salt-free bouillon powder

1. Sieve the peas and rinse well under cold water. Put them in a pan with 1.5 ltr water.
2. Bring to the boil and skim off the excess foam.
3. Add the sweet potato, carrots, onion and bouillon.
4. Boil for 10 minutes, lower the heat then simmer for another 15 minutes.
5. Blend until smooth, or blend half of the soup then mix it back in with the half you didn't blend – this makes it more chunky.
6. Pour into warmed bowls, toss a handful of fresh, raw alfalfa sprouts into each bowl and serve immediately.

Oriental Style Salad
SERVES 1
1 courgette
1/2 cucumber
1/2 red or yellow pepper
1 carrot
2 spring onions, sliced
beansprouts
green salad leaves
FOR THE DRESSING
1 tbsp wheat-free Tamari sauce
1 tsp sesame oil
2 tbsp water
1 clove garlic, crushed

1. Cut the courgettes, cucumber, peppers and carrots into long thin sticks.
2. Toss with sliced spring onions and rinsed beansprouts.
3. Mix together Tamari sauce, sesame oil, water and garlic.
4. Drizzle the dressing over the salad.
5. Serve over green salad leaves.

Cucumbers are a fabulous food for weight loss and a perfect anti-bloat food because of their diuretic properties. So don't scoff at them, just eat them and make lots of juices with them too.

Day6

BREAKFAST

1 cup of warm water with a squeeze of lemon
1 cup of Dandelion tea
followed by a smoothie.

Plummy Fruit Smoothie
This smoothie is also delicious with
a few berries added to the blend.

SERVES 1
3 plums
3 nectarines
3 ripe pears
200ml water

Blend all ingredients until smooth
and creamy

**REMEMBER TO SOAK YOUR MUNG BEANS
FOR DINNER TONIGHT.**

MID-MORNING SNACK
One ripe banana.

LUNCH

**Easy Peasy Yellow Pea Soup (from
last night) with Avocado and Salad.**
Sprinkle your soup with raw shelled hemp
seeds and/or sprouted alfalfa seeds.

Avocado
One ripe avocado, halved and stoned.

Purple Sprouting Broccoli Salad
with Radish
The pistachio nuts add a lovely crunch
to this salad but if you are seriously trying
for weight loss then I would advise that
you omit them at this time.

SERVES 1
75g well trimmed purple sprouting broccoli
30g fresh radish, sliced
25g shelled peas
1/2 tbsp mirin
1 1/2 tbsp wheat-free Tamari sauce
1 tbsp pistachio nuts (optional)

1. Cut the broccoli in half lengthways and
then into bite-sized pieces, then arrange
on a salad plate.
2. Scatter over the radish and peas then
sprinkle with the mirin and Tamari.
3. Add the nuts and serve immediately.

MID-AFTERNOON SNACK
**Four chicory leaves, topped with houmous
and baby tomatoes.**

DINNER

Gourmet Mighty Mung Bean Casserole served with brown rice and salad.

Gourmet Mighty Mung Bean Casserole

Reserve a portion for your lunch tomorrow.

SERVES 4–6

250g mung beans, soaked in 1 ltr cold
water for 6 hours
1 ltr water or vegetable stock
1 tsp fennel seeds
180g celeriac, peeled and diced
100g celery, chopped
150g leeks, chopped
2 small Bok Choy
watercress or rocket

1. Drain the mung beans and rinse well.
2. Bring the water or stock to the boil, add the beans and simmer for 10 minutes. Skim away any white scum that rises to the surface.
3. Add the fennel seeds and celeriac and simmer for 10 minutes.
4. Add the celery and leeks and simmer for a further 10 minutes.
5. Remove from the heat. Stir in the Bok Choy, put in warmed bowls and sprinkle with the watercress or rocket.
6. Serve with a simple green leafy salad and brown rice.

The Mighty Mung Bean – my anti-toxin. I rave about the mung bean, as many of you probably know. They cook very quickly and are super easy to digest. I use mung beans to purge the body of toxins or excess acids caused by poor diets. And mung beans release energy steadily, keeping blood sugar balanced.

Day 7

BREAKFAST

1 cup of warm water with squeeze of lemon
1 cup of Dandelion tea
followed by a smoothie.

Tangy Smoothie
SERVES 1
1/2 pineapple
1 mango
1 banana
1 plum

Blend all ingredients until smooth and creamy.

MID-MORNING SNACK
One or more apples.

LUNCH
Mung Bean Salad made from Gourmet Mighty Mung Bean Casserole.

Mung Bean Salad
SERVES 1
1 portion of Gourmet Mighty Mung Bean Casserole, and any left over brown rice
60g radish
3 spring onions
1 tbsp lemon juice
50g fresh rocket
2 tbsps raw shelled hemp seeds (optional)

1. Drain any excess moisture from the beans.
2. Place in a mixing bowl with all the other ingredients and toss them together.
3. Serve immediately.

MID-AFTERNOON SNACK
Veggie Juice or a handful of salt-free hazelnuts (organic if possible).

Veggie Juice
SERVES 1
handful of spinach
6 carrots
3 celery stalks

DINNER
Baked White Fish with Minted Mushy Peas on a bed of salad.

Baked White Fish with Minted Mushy Peas

Any white fish works well in this recipe, whiting, haddock or cod, for example. This is a great fast meal to make when you get in from work.

SERVES 4
1 tsp oil
4 100g skinless white fish fillets
1 lemon, sliced
2 cloves garlic, peeled and sliced
a few sprigs of dill or fennel
125g new season or frozen peas
a large sprig of fresh mint
1 tsp mirin

1. Preheat the oven to 200C/Gas 6.
2. Take a large piece of foil and, with a pastry brush, oil the centre. Place the fish on the foil and cover with the lemon slices and garlic. Scatter over the dill or fennel. Scrunch up the foil to make a parcel and place on a baking tray.

3. Place in the oven and cook for 6–7 minutes. Remove from the oven and allow to stand for 10 minutes.
4. Bring a small pan of water to the boil and add the mint and peas and cook (fresh peas for 1–2 minutes, frozen for 30 seconds). Remove from the heat and drain.
5. Place the peas in a small bowl with the mirin and mash with a fork.
6. Divide the peas and fish between 4 warmed serving plates and serve immediately with some raw green salad leaves.

SOAK 1 CUP OF BUCKWHEAT OVERNIGHT FOR YOUR MORNING PORRIDGE. THIS WAY YOUR PORRIDGE WILL BE READY IN NO TIME.

Look at yourself in a mirror right now. See and envision the possibilities of who you can truly be when you set your mind to it.

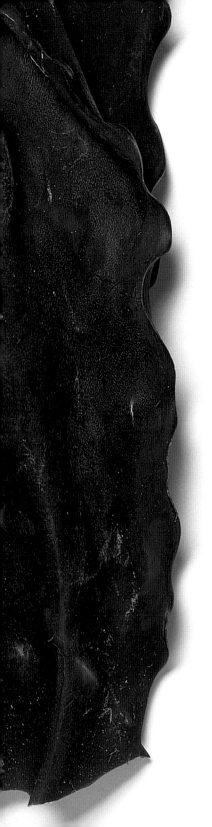

Day 8

BREAKFAST

1 cup of warm water
1 cup of Dandelion tea
followed by 1 large grapefruit and Buckwheat
Cinnamon Porridge.

Buckwheat Cinnamon Porridge
SERVES 1–2
125g buckwheat groats
1 tsp lemon zest and a squeeze of lemon juice
**1cm piece fresh ginger root, peeled and
grated**
1 cinnamon stick, broken
**raw shelled hemp seeds or sunflower seeds
(optional)**

1. Place the buckwheat, lemon zest and
juice, ginger, cinnamon and 500ml of water
in a pan. Bring to the boil, then lower the
heat and simmer for 20 minutes.
2. Serve with a sprinkling of sunflower
or shelled hemp seeds.

MID-MORNING SNACK
Punnets of berries (choose from strawberries,
gooseberries, blackberries or blueberries).

My Dad introduced me
to grapefruit for breakfast
as a child. I am glad he
was a grapefruit fanatic
as they are packed with
antioxidants.

LUNCH
Haricot Bean Salad.

Haricot Bean Salad
SERVES 2
1 can no salt, no sugar haricot beans
1/2 red onion, finely chopped
1 clove garlic, crushed
1 tbsp fresh parsley, chopped
2 tbsps extra virgin olive oil
2 tsps apple cider vinegar
1 small bag mixed leaf and herb salad
1 chicory, sliced
1 red pepper, finely diced
8–10 green beans

1. Drain the haricot beans and rinse under cold water.
2. Put the beans, red onion, garlic, parsley, olive oil and cider vinegar in a bowl, toss together then set aside for 10 minutes.
3. Cook the green beans in boiling water for 2–3 minutes, then plunge into cold water to cool.
4. Empty the mixed leaf and herb salad into a bowl. Add the chicory, red pepper and cooled green beans.
5. Spoon the haricot beans with dressing over the salad and serve.

MID-AFTERNOON SNACK
Vegetable crudités (four radish and one yellow pepper, chopped) and dip (see page 200 for dips).

DINNER
Fresh vegetable juice followed by baked squash with mashed avocado and beansprout topping.

Veggie Juice
C'mon you can do it. It'll take you two minutes. If you don't manage a veggie juice during the day, it's a fantastic pick-me-up for when you come home from work.

SERVES 1
4–5 carrots
1 cucumber
1 stick of celery

Juice all ingredients and drink slowly.

Baked Squash
Pop a squash in the oven and let it bake while you drink your juice.

Topping
You can add any fresh raw vegetables to this mix, just mash them all in there.

SERVES 1
1 avocado
fresh dill
generous portion of beansprouts
generous portion of alfalfa sprouts
2 radishes, sliced
lemon juice

1. Mash the avocado with the dill, beansprouts and alfalfa sprouts.
2. Squeeze some lemon juice over the top and add a couple of radishes for garnish.
3. Pile on top of baked squash and serve.

Day 9

BREAKFAST

1 cup of warm water
1 cup of Dandelion tea
followed by fruit salad.

Fruit Salad
SERVES 1
1 banana
1/2 small tub blueberries
1 peach
1/2 small tub raspberries or strawberries

MID-MORNING SNACK
A cup of instant miso soup. Add four chopped radish for a crunchy texture.

LUNCH
Risotto of Fennel and Broad Beans.

Risotto of Fennel and Broad Beans
SERVES 1
1 small onion, finely chopped
1/2 fennel bulb, core removed, finely chopped
2 cloves garlic, chopped
2 tsps olive oil
1 tbsp water
100g brown rice
250ml vegetable stock
75g baby broad beans
2 tbsps freshly chopped chervil

1. Place the onion, fennel, garlic, oil and water in a non-stick pan and cook gently for 5 minutes.
2. Add the rice and stir well.
3. Gradually add the stock, 1 ladleful at a time, and cook until the rice is tender – about 15–20 minutes.
4. Stir in the broad beans and chervil and serve immediately.

MID-AFTERNOON SNACK
Small bowl of cherry tomatoes or baby plum tomatoes.

Miso is one of the most valuable healing foods and I want you to try it. It's made from fermented soybean paste and it has a unique nutritional profile packed with easy to digest protein and energy boosting vitamins. You can find it in powder or paste form in the health food store. Use miso in your cooking instead of plain old table salt and reap a variety of benefits in addition to enhanced flavour.

DINNER

Soup, followed by Baked Salmon served with steamed vegetables.

5 Minute Soup

Save a portion for your lunch tomorrow.

SERVES 1–2
500ml water
1 clove garlic
small piece of fresh root ginger, peeled and finely sliced
1/2 225g-slab of firm tofu, cut into small squares
8 mangetout, trimmed and finely sliced lengthways
1 small red pepper, de-seeded and cut into short thin strips
small handful of fresh or frozen peas
1 Bok Choy, leaves separated, washed and sliced
2 spring onions, trimmed and sliced
2 sachets of instant miso soup (robust flavour)
handful of alfalfa sprouts
fresh coriander to garnish

1. Bring the water to the boil in a large saucepan, add the garlic and ginger and boil for 1 minute.
2. Stir in the tofu, mangetout, pepper and peas. Return to the boil, skim any foam from the surface with a spoon, and simmer for 2 minutes.
3. Add the Bok Choy and spring onions and cook for 1 minute.
4. Remove from the heat and stir in the miso soup and beansprouts.
5. Ladle into a warmed bowl to serve. Garnish with fresh chopped coriander.

Simple Baked Salmon

SERVES 1
boneless fillet of salmon
small head of broccoli
2 carrots, cut into batons
lemon and lime wedges to serve
salad leaves (optional)

1. Heat the oven to 200C/Gas 6.
2. Place the salmon on a baking tray and cook in the oven for 18–20 minutes until cooked through.
3. Steam the carrots for a few minutes then add the broccoli and lightly cook.
4. Place the carrots and broccoli on a plate and lay the salmon fillet on top. Add a couple of lime and lemon wedges for squeezing over the fish.
5. Serve with some raw salad leaves if you like.

PUT 100G ADZUKI BEANS IN A BOWL WITH PLENTY OF COLD WATER AND LEAVE THEM IN THE FRIDGE TO SOAK OVERNIGHT (FOR DINNER TOMORROW).

Day 10

BREAKFAST

1 cup of warm water
1 cup Fennel tea
followed by Stewed Apples.

Stewed Apples over Fresh Blueberries

Fresh raspberries also work well with
stewed apple. My favourite stewing apples
are Bramleys.

SERVES 1
2 apples
250ml water
squeeze lemon juice
1 pear, chopped
1 tub blueberries

1. Chop the apples, put them in a pan
with the water and lemon juice, and
stew until soft.
2. Serve over the chopped pear
and blueberries.

MID-MORNING SNACK

Two papayas or two nectarines.

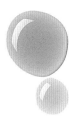

LUNCH

**5 Minute Soup from yesterday, followed by Fresh Tuna
with Steamed Kale and Caper Dressing.**

Fresh Tuna with Steamed Kale and Caper Dressing

In this recipe you could use crushed
chickpeas flavoured with a little brown
rice vinegar instead of the avocado, and
use parsley rather than capers.

SERVES 1
150g tuna steak
150g fresh kale
1 avocado, peeled and stone removed
FOR THE DRESSING
3 tbsps capers
2–3 tbsps fresh parsley
juice of 1 lemon, plus a little extra
1 tsp oil
3 tbsps hot water

1. Heat a non-stick pan and cook the tuna
for 2–3 minutes on each side.
2. Remove the tuna from the pan. Add the
kale to the pan with 1 tbsp water and cook
for 2 minutes, or until just wilted.
3. Mix the capers, parsley, lemon juice,
oil and hot water together and whisk well.
4. Crush the avocado with a little lemon
juice, using the back of a fork.
5. Place the avocado on a serving plate and
arrange the kale around it. Place the tuna
on the avocado.
6. Spoon over half the dressing (reserve
the rest for a salad tomorrow) and serve
immediately.

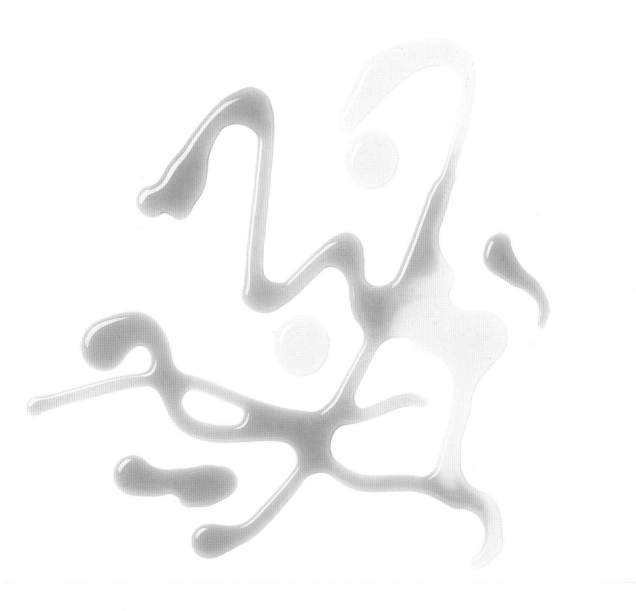

MID-AFTERNOON SNACK
Veggie Juice or half a cucumber, finely chopped.

Veggie Juice
SERVES 1
**1 cucumber
2 celery stalks
handful alfalfa sprouts
tiny piece of ginger**

DINNER
Adzuki Bean Hotpot served with Crunchy Green Salad.

Adzuki Bean Hotpot
The fresher the beans the quicker they will cook, but there is no way of telling how fresh they are when you buy them. So be prepared to cook the beans for longer if necessary and add extra water if they appear to be drying out. Reserve a portion for your lunch tomorrow.

SERVES 4
**100g dried adzuki beans, soaked and rinsed
1.75 ltrs cold water
1 tbsp extra virgin olive oil
1 medium onion, peeled and chopped
2 garlic cloves, peeled and crushed
1 celery stick, trimmed and sliced
3 medium carrots, peeled and sliced
1 large parsnip, peeled and cubed
1 large sweet potato, peeled and cubed
(around 400g prepared weight)
400-g can chopped tomatoes
1/2 organic wheat-free stock cube
2 medium leeks, trimmed and sliced**

1. Place the beans in a bowl to soak, cover with plenty of cold water and leave in the fridge overnight. Drain well.

2. Place the soaked beans in a large saucepan. Cover with 1.75 ltrs cold water and bring to the boil. Boil hard for 15 minutes, then reduce the heat slightly and simmer for a further 30–40 minutes until the beans are tender, stirring occasionally. Add an extra cup or two of water if the beans begin to look dry.

3. While the beans are cooking, heat the oil in a large saucepan or flame-proof casserole and very gently cook the onion, garlic and celery for 5 minutes until well softened but not coloured, stirring regularly.

4. Add the carrots, parsnip and sweet potato to the pan. Cook gently for 10 minutes, stirring occasionally.

5. Stir in the canned tomatoes. Half fill the empty can with water and pour over the vegetables.

6. Add the half stock cube and bring to the boil. Reduce the heat slightly and simmer for 5 minutes.

7. Add the leeks and continue to simmer for 10–15 minutes more until all the vegetables are just tender and the sauce is thick.

8. Drain the cooked adzuki beans in a colander and stir into the vegetable mixture.

9. Spoon the adzuki bean mixture into a 2-litre/4-pint ovenproof dish. Bake in a preheated oven at 200C/Gas 6 for 20 minutes.

10. Serve with Crunchy Green Salad.

Crunchy Green Salad

SERVES 3–4

1 large handful fine green beans, trimmed
150g pack asparagus tips, trimmed
150g pack tenderstem broccoli, trimmed and broken into thin lengths
4 tbsp fresh or frozen peas
1 fennel bulb, trimmed and finely sliced
2 celery sticks, trimmed and sliced
1 little gem lettuce, trimmed and thickly sliced
3 tbsp pine nuts
3 tbsp pumpkin seeds

FOR THE DRESSING
4 tbsp extra virgin olive oil
1 tbsp freshly squeezed lemon juice
1 garlic clove, peeled and crushed

1. Bring a large pan of water to the boil. Add the green beans, return to the boil and cook for 2 minutes.

2. Add the asparagus, tenderstem broccoli and peas. Return to the boil and cook for just one minute. Drain the beans and asparagus in a colander and rinse under running water until cold. Transfer to a serving dish.

3. Toss the fennel, celery, little gem lettuce, pine nuts and pumpkin seeds with the blanched vegetables.

4. Whisk the oil, lemon juice and garlic together with a fork and pour over the salad just before serving.

Day 11

BREAKFAST

1 cup of warm water
1 cup Slippery Elm tea
followed by fruit salad.

Fruit Salad
SERVES 1
1 apple
2 peaches
1 pear
1 banana

MID-MORNING SNACK
Juice of two whole pink grapefruit.

LUNCH
Adzuki Bean Hot Pot from yesterday, served with salad.

Mangetout and Sauerkraut Salad
SERVES 1
6 mangetout
4 chicory leaves
1 tbsp sauerkraut
1 little gem lettuce, shredded
squeeze of lemon juice
2 tsp hemp oil
2 lightly steamed asparagus (optional),
finely chopped

1. Arrange the raw ingredients in an artistic way on a large plate.
2. Drizzle the hemp oil over the salad and top with a squeeze of lemon and the asparagus.

MID-AFTERNOON SNACK
Handful of unsalted cashew nuts and handful of sunflower/pumpkin seeds.

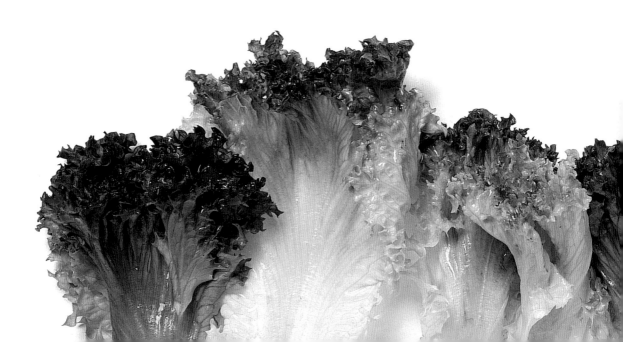

DINNER

Soup followed by Butter Bean Spread with vegetable crudités.

Courgette Soup

Reserve a portion for lunch tomorrow.

SERVES 4
600g courgettes, sliced
2 onions, chopped
750ml water
1 tbsp fresh chives, chopped

1. Place the courgettes, onion and 2 tbsp of the water in a non-stick saucepan and cook over a gentle heat for 5–10 minutes to soften but not colour.
2. Add the remaining water, bring to the boil and simmer for 5 minutes.
3. Remove from the heat, allow to cool slightly and then blend in a food processor or blender.
4. Spoon into warm bowls, sprinkle with chives and serve.

Butter Bean Spread

This is also good used as a topping for baked vegetables.

1 can organic butter beans
1/2 small onion, chopped
1 garlic bulb, peeled and chopped
2 tbsps chopped fresh parsley
2 tbsps chopped fresh dill
1 tbsp Tahini
2 tsps miso paste
1 small garlic clove, peeled and chopped

1. Place all the ingredients in a food processor and blend until smooth.
2. Serve with fresh vegetable crudités of your choice.

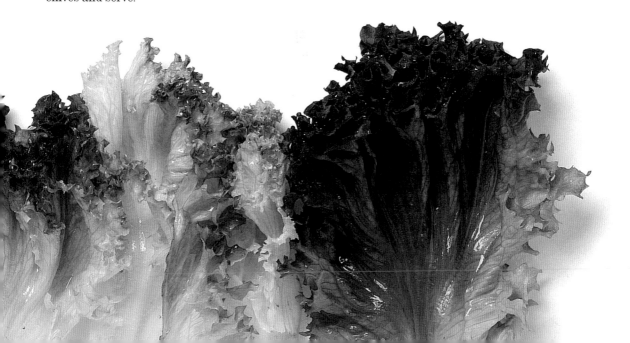

Day 12

BREAKFAST

1 cup of warm water
1 cup of Nettle or Dandelion tea
followed by vegetable juice.

Vegetable Juice
SERVES 1
6 carrots
1 stick of celery
1/2 beetroot
1 cucumber

Push all the ingredients through
a juicer and drink slowly.

MID-MORNING SNACK
One mango with a handful of raspberries.

LUNCH
Courgette Soup from yesterday, followed by salad.

Quickest Quinoa Salad
SERVES 1
50g quinoa grain
small bag of mixed salad leaves
enough of each of the following to your
taste to make a good sized bowl of salad:
cucumber
beetroot, cooked
spring onions, sliced
chicory, sliced
mangetout
parsley, chopped
hazelnuts (optional)

1. Rinse the quinoa then cook in boiling
water for 10 minutes until tender. Drain
in a sieve under cold running water.
2. Cut the cucumber into cubes, the beetroot
into wedges, and toss in a bowl with the
quinoa, spring onions, chicory, washed
and trimmed mangetout and the parsley.
3. Serve on a bed of mixed salad leaves
and sprinkle with hazelnuts.

IF YOU WANT A FANCY OPTION
Place the spring onions in a mixture of 1 tbsp
umeboshi vinegar and 1 1/2 tbsp brown rice
vinegar an hour before preparing your salad.
Mix in with the quinoa salad, and add 3 raw
radishes before serving.

This option is not really necessary but
I just want you to be thinking ahead about
what you can do with food for a day when you
might want to experiment. You could add
onion to pickle too if you want to get fancy.

MID-AFTERNOON SNACK
Handful of mixed seeds.

DINNER

Haddock with Braised Fennel
A simple fish dish as an alternative to
the fish burger when you are in a hurry.
It contains the spice star anise which
is good for flu-fighting.

SERVES 4
4 100g skinless haddock fillets
2 fennel bulbs, finely sliced, core removed
2 star anise
200ml cold water
1 lemon, sliced
1 tbsp black olives (optional)

1. Preheat the oven to 180C/Gas 4.
2. Place the fennel in a baking dish or
roasting pan, add the star anise and water
and bake for 15 minutes.
3. Remove the pan from the oven and lay the
fish on the fennel. Arrange the lemon slices
on the fish then return it to the oven and
bake for a further 7–10 minutes.
4. Remove the pan from the oven and allow
to stand for 5 minutes. Scatter with olives
and serve immediately.

REMEMBER TO LEAVE YOUR BLACK TURTLE BEANS
TO SOAK OVERNIGHT IN PLENTY OF WATER READY
FOR TOMORROW.

Nothing beats the taste
of a freshly blended
veggie juice. Freshly made
vegetable juices are a
potent source of nutrients
and if you drink them on
a regular basis you'll enjoy
clearer skin, better energy
levels and balanced
overall health.

Day 13

BREAKFAST

1 cup of warm water
1 cup of Slippery Elm tea
followed by a smoothie.

Strawberry and Peach Smoothie
SERVES 1
1 small punnet strawberries
2 peaches, stoned and chopped
1 banana
1 pear, finely chopped

1. Blend the strawberries, peaches and banana until smooth.
2. Pour over the chopped pear and serve.

MID-MORNING SNACK
Bowl of grapes.

LUNCH
Quinoa and Beetroot Salad.

Quinoa and Beetroot Salad
SERVES 2–3
100g quinoa grain, rinsed
100g green beans, trimmed and cut into 2cm lengths
75g cucumber, halved lengthways and thinly sliced
2 vacuum-packed beetroot (no vinegar or sugar), drained and cut into thin wedges
1 spring onion, trimmed and thinly sliced
1/2 small yellow pepper, de-seeded and thinly sliced
5 cherry tomatoes, halved
2 tbsp olive oil
2 tbsp freshly squeezed lemon juice
1 garlic clove, peeled and crushed
2 tbsp finely chopped fresh parsley

1. Cook the quinoa in a pan of boiling water for 12–15 minutes, or as instructed on the packet, until tender.
2. Cook the beans in a small pan of boiling water for 4 minutes until tender-crisp.
3. Drain the quinoa in a sieve under running water until cold. Press with the back of a spoon to remove the excess water. Tip into a serving bowl.
4. Drain the beans under running water until cold and add to the quinoa.
5. Add all the remaining ingredients and toss well together. Set aside for at least 15 minutes to allow the flavours to develop, then serve.

MID-AFTERNOON SNACK
Four baby radish and a handful of Brazil nuts.

DINNER
Black Bean Soup with Avocado Drizzle and Wild Rocket.

Black Bean Soup with Avocado Drizzle and Wild Rocket

This Mexican style soup is packed with flavour and makes a very satisfying supper dish. The black bean soup contrasts well in both colour and taste with the avocado salsa.

SERVES 4

250g Black Turtle beans, soaked overnight
1 onion, finely chopped
2 cloves garlic, peeled
1 leek, finely sliced
2 tbsp water
1 tsp olive oil
1 red pepper, finely chopped
1 ltr water or homemade stock
1 tsp coriander seeds, roughly ground
2 tbsp fresh parsley
4 tbsp fresh coriander, finely chopped
1 ripe avocado, peeled, stoned and finely chopped
1/2 red onion, finely chopped
juice of 1 lime
50g rocket, roughly torn or chopped

1. Soak the beans in cold water overnight. Drain and rinse well.
2. Place the onion, garlic, leek, water and oil in a non-stick casserole dish, cover and cook over a low heat for 3–4 minutes until soft.
3. Add the water or stock, and the pepper. Bring to the boil and add the coriander seeds, parsley, fresh coriander and the beans. Simmer for 35–40 minutes.
4. Place the avocado and red onion in a small bowl with the lime juice and the rocket, stir gently to mix but not to mush the avocado.
5. Remove the soup from the heat and allow to cool slightly. Transfer half the soup to the processor and process until smooth. Return the processed soup to the pan, stir to mix the two soups and reheat gently.
6. Place a large spoonful of the avocado mixture in the centre of four shallow bowls. Spoon the warmed soup around the avocado and serve immediately.

The Queen of Grains, quinoa is a fantastic source of protein, containing all the essential amino acids. Quinoa is your kidney supporter. And I consider your kidneys to be your bank account for life, so add interest with quinoa porridges, quinoa salads and even my favourite, quinoa in soups.

Day 14

BREAKFAST

1 cup of warm water
1 cup of Nettle tea
followed by fruit salad and a bowl
of Easy Oats.

Fruit Berry Salad
SERVES 1
1 small tub blueberries
1 small tub raspberries
1 small punnet strawberries

Easy Oats

If you are still hungry, you can have
a bowl of porridge oats, but you need to
wait 20 minutes to let your fruit digest.

SERVES 1
100g porridge oats
400ml water or rice milk

1. Combine the porridge oats with
the water or rice milk in a pan.
2. Bring to the boil, then lower the heat
and simmer for 15–20 minutes.
3. Season with a sprinkle of cinnamon.

MID-MORNING SNACK
Bowl of mung bean sprouts with a sprinkle of raw
shelled hemp, pumpkin or sunflower seeds.

LUNCH
Black Bean Soup with Avocado Salsa from yesterday,
with some chopped raw chicory leaves.

MID-AFTERNOON SNACK
Chop up a courgette and top with houmous
and shredded carrot.

I want you to try every food
I put before you even if you
have never tried it before.
I need you to go beyond
your comfort zone of foods
that you usually eat. Also,
just because you don't love
something the first time
you try it does not mean
that you won't like it in the
future. Keep an open mind.

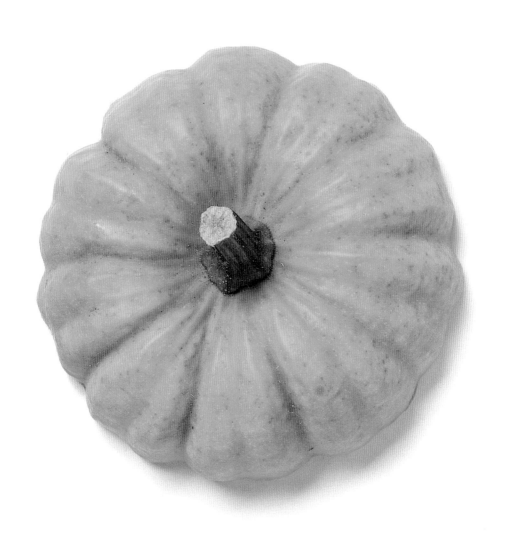

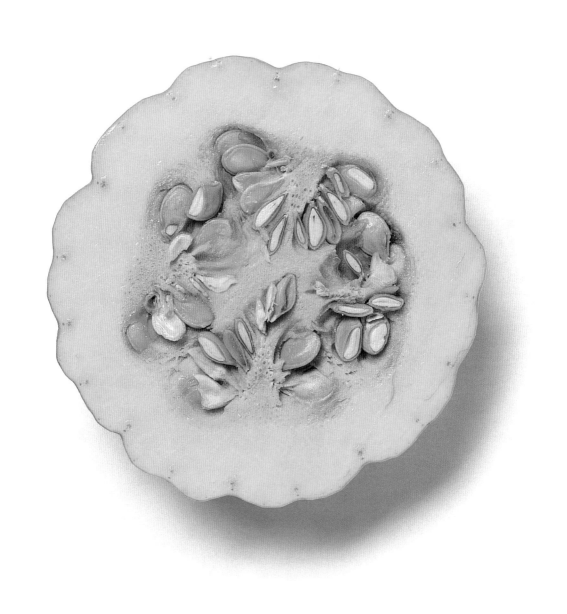

DINNER
Lemony Chicken Burgers served with a leafy green salad, or Tempeh Cutlets.

Lemony Chicken Burgers
Reserve two burgers for the following day. Allow them to cool then cover and chill.

MAKES 6 BURGERS
2 tsp cold-pressed sunflower oil, plus extra for greasing
50g onion, finely chopped
1 slim leek, trimmed and chopped
1 garlic clove, peeled and crushed
2 skinless, boneless free-range or organic chicken breasts (about 350g)
1/2 tsp organic wheat-free vegetable bouillon powder
1 tbsp freshly squeezed lemon juice
finely grated zest of a small lemon

1. Gently heat the oil in a pan with a little water and cook the onion, leek and garlic over a low heat for 2 minutes until softened but not coloured, stirring occasionally. Set aside to cool.
2. Preheat the oven to 200C/Gas 6. Lightly oil a baking tray. Cut the chicken breasts into chunks and place in a food processor. Blend until fairly finely chopped but not mushy – you may have to remove the lid and push the chicken down once or twice until the right consistency is reached.
3. Transfer the chicken to a bowl and stir in the cooked onion, leek and garlic, bouillon powder, lemon juice and zest. Mix well with clean hands and form into six balls.
4. Place the balls, evenly spaced apart, on the baking tray and flatten into burger shapes.
5. Bake for 10 minutes then remove from the oven and turn over. Brush with a little more oil and return to the oven for a further 5 minutes until cooked through.
6. Serve hot or cold with a large mixed salad.

Tempeh Cutlets
SERVES 4
225g tempeh
large piece ginger, sliced into 9 pieces
125g watercress leaves
125g beansprouts
50g Daikon radish, cut into fine julienne
1 tsp sesame oil
3 tbsp water
dash of wheat-free Tamari sauce

1. Arrange the ginger slices over the top of the tempeh.
2. Place the tempeh in a steamer basket over a pan of hot water, or in an electric steamer. Steam for 10 minutes.
3. Discard the ginger and slice the tempeh into 1 1/2 cm slices.
4. Arrange the watercress, beansprouts and Daikon on four serving plates.
5. Heat the sesame oil and water in a non-stick frying pan. Add the tempeh slices, cut side down, and water-fry for 1 minute. Turn the tempeh over and sprinkle with a little Tamari sauce and cook for a further minute.
6. Arrange the tempeh slices on the salad bed and spoon over a little of the cooking liquid. Serve immediately.

Day 15

BREAKFAST

1 cup of warm water
1 cup of Sage herbal tea
followed by fruit salad.

Fruit Salad
SERVES 1
1 mango, stoned and chopped
1 banana
2 peaches, stoned and chopped
1/2 small tub blueberries
1/2 small tub raspberries

MID-MORNING SNACK
Juice of two apples and two pears.

Imagine what it's like to feel absolutely fantastic. That can easily be you.

LUNCH
Cashew Chicken Salad made with Chicken Burgers from yesterday; or Cashew Tofu Salad.

Cashew Chicken or Cashew Tofu Salad
For the vegetarian alternative, substitute tofu for the chicken. My salad is great for packed lunches and can be prepared the night before. Simply cool the vegetables before adding the rest of the ingredients, then cover and chill.

SERVES 2
1 tbsp olive oil
1 red pepper, cut into 2cm pieces
75g mangetout, trimmed
1 tsp wheat-free Tamari sauce
2 cooked Lemony Chicken Burgers
OR 75g firm tofu cut into small squares
2 spring onions, trimmed and sliced
10g plain cashew nuts, roughly chopped
1 romaine lettuce heart, leaves separated, washed and drained
extra virgin olive oil and Tamari sauce, to serve

1. Heat the oil in a large wok with a little water. Sauté the pepper over a medium heat for 2 minutes.
2. Add the mangetout and sauté for 30 seconds. Remove from the heat and sprinkle with the Tamari sauce.
3. Arrange the lettuce leaves in two bowls – tearing in half first if the leaves are large. Scatter the pepper and mangetout over the lettuce.
4. Slice the chicken burgers and arrange on top. Or if making tofu version, arrange tofu squares on top. Sprinkle with the spring onions and nuts.
5. Drizzle with a little olive oil and extra Tamari sauce to serve.

MID-AFTERNOON SNACK

Veggie Juice or steamed corn on the cob spread with a little umeboshi plum sauce.

Veggie Juice
SERVES 1
6 carrots
2 celery stalks
4 sprigs parsley

DINNER

Gentle Lentil Curry with Tomato and Coriander Relish.

Gentle Lentil Curry

Reserve a portion for lunch tomorrow.

SERVES 4
1 tbsp olive oil
1 medium onion, peeled and chopped
2 garlic cloves, peeled and crushed
1 tsp ground cumin
1/2 tsp ground turmeric
1/2 tsp ground ginger
150g split red lentils, washed and drained
2 medium carrots, peeled and sliced
1 medium sweet potato, peeled and cut
into 2cm chunks
900ml cold water
75g green beans, trimmed and cut into
2cm lengths
75g frozen peas
sauerkraut (optional)
freshly cooked brown rice, to serve (optional)

1. Heat the oil in a large saucepan and cook the onion and garlic over a low heat for 3 minutes until softened but not coloured.

2. Add the cumin, turmeric and ginger and cook for 2 minutes, stirring regularly.
3. Stir in the lentils, carrots and sweet potato. Turn in the oil for a few seconds then add the cold water.
4. Bring to the boil and skim off any foam that rises to the surface. Boil for about 12–15 minutes until the lentils start to soften.
5. Add the beans and peas and continue to cook for 5 minutes more, stirring occasionally until the lentils are very soft and the vegetables are tender. Stir regularly, especially towards the end of the cooking time.
6. Serve with Tomato and Coriander Relish, sauerkraut and freshly cooked brown rice if liked.

Tomato and Coriander Relish
SERVES 2
2 vine-ripened tomatoes, roughly chopped
2 spring onions, trimmed and finely sliced
2 tbsp chopped fresh coriander
1 tbsp freshly squeezed lime juice

Mix all the ingredients in a small bowl and leave for at least 30 minutes before serving.

Day 16

BREAKFAST

1 cup of warm water
1 cup Dandelion tea
followed by a smoothie.

Soft Fruit Smoothie
SERVES 1
1 nectarine
1 soft pear
1 peach
1 tub berries

1. Blend until smooth.
2. You can always add a little pressed apple juice if this is too thick to blend.

MID-MORNING SNACK
Two celery stalks and half a cucumber, finely chopped. Serve with a dip if you fancy (see page 200).

LUNCH
Gentle Lentil Soup made with Gentle Lentil Curry from the day before.

Gentle Lentil Soup
SERVES 1
Reserved portion of Gentle Lentil Curry
300ml water or stock

Simply put the curry and water in a food processor and blend until smooth. If you prefer a thicker or thinner soup add less or more water accordingly.

MID-AFTERNOON SNACK
Veggie Juice or one yellow pepper, sliced.

Veggie Juice
SERVES 1
6 carrots
1 cucumber
1 celery stalk
handful parsley
tiny piece of ginger

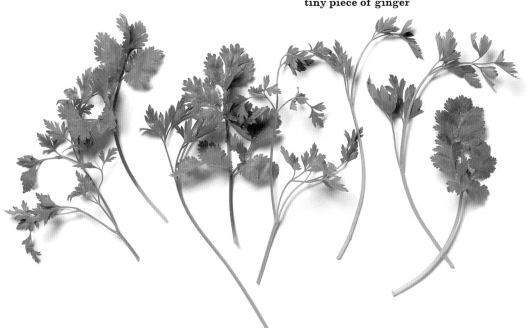

DINNER
Sushi Wraps.

Sushi Wraps

Wasabi paste (optional) can be purchased from oriental groceries and health food shops in small tubes. It adds a little extra to the avocado and chickpea paste, but it is not essential. Sushi Daikon comes vacuum packed from the same sources and once opened keeps well in the fridge. Reserve enough sushi for lunch the next day, wrapping the rolls in cling film and storing them in the fridge.

SERVES 2–3
100g short grain brown rice
1 tsp brown rice vinegar
1 avocado, peeled and stoned
220g chickpeas drained
2.5cm wasabi paste (optional)
plus additional to serve
juice of half a lemon
19g toasted Nori seaweed sheets (7 pieces)
3 sticks of celery, peeled and cut into fine strips
2 carrots, peeled and cut into fine strips
20g sushi Daikon (or radish)
pickled ginger (or raw ginger)
wheat-free soy sauce

1. Place the rice in a small pan and cover with 250ml water. Bring to the boil, cover and simmer for 5 minutes.

2. Remove the pan from the heat and leave to stand for 15 minutes. Drain the rice in a colander.

3. Transfer the rice to a bowl, add the vinegar and mix well.

4. Place the avocado, chickpeas and wasabi (optional) in the food processor, process for 30 seconds then add the lemon juice and process for a few more seconds.

5. Place a seaweed wrap on a clean working board. Spread a thin layer of the avocado mixture over the seaweed and cover with a layer of rice. Place a line of celery and carrot down the centre of the rice.

6. Carefully roll up the sushi, and roll backward and forward a couple of times to tighten the roll. Place on a plate in the fridge and leave to chill for 5 minutes, repeat the process with the remaining ingredients.

7. Slice the sushi rolls into 2cm pieces. Serve with additional wasabi mustard, pickled ginger and wheat-free soy sauce to taste.

Seaweeds are packed full of minerals, including calcium. I believe that low levels of dietary minerals are at epidemic levels in this country, so get into seaweeds to soak up more minerals.

Day 17

BREAKFAST

1 cup of warm water
1 cup Nettle tea
followed by a smoothie.

Berry Delight
SERVES 1
1 small punnet strawberries
2 soft pears
1 banana
100ml water

Blend until smooth.

MID-MORNING SNACK
Bowl of grapes.

LUNCH
Sushi Wraps from yesterday, served with salad.

Oriental Style Salad
SERVES 1
1 courgettes
1/2 cucumber
1/2 red or yellow pepper
1 carrots
2 spring onions, sliced
beansprouts
green salad leaves
FOR THE DRESSING
1 tbsp wheat-free Tamari sauce
1 tsp sesame oil
2 tbsp water
1 clove garlic, crushed

1. Cut the courgettes, cucumber, peppers and carrots into long thin sticks.
2. Toss with sliced spring onions and rinsed beansprouts.
3. Mix together Tamari sauce, sesame oil, water and garlic.
4. Drizzle the dressing over the salad.
5. Serve over green salad leaves.

MID-AFTERNOON SNACK
One ripe avocado with a sprinkle of raw shelled hemp seeds and a teaspoon of houmous.

DINNER
Quick Cabbage and Bean Stew.

Quick Cabbage and Bean Stew
SERVES 2

1 onion, sliced
2 cloves garlic, crushed
3 carrots, peeled and sliced
1 sweet potato, peeled and diced
1 organic, wheat-free veggie stock cube
or 1 tbsp miso paste
1.25 ltrs cold water
1/2 small Savoy cabbage
400-g can haricot beans
2 tbsp parsley, chopped

1. Place the onion, garlic, carrots, sweet potato, miso or stock, and 1.25 ltrs cold water in a pan. Bring to the boil.
2. Drain and rinse the haricot beans.
3. Stir in the shredded cabbage, beans and parsley.
4. Return to the boil and simmer until the cabbage is tender.

Eat cruciferous veggies as much as you can. Eat them raw and eat them cooked too. Vary the way you prepare them. Cabbage, broccoli, Brussels sprouts, turnip greens, watercress and kale have been found to have potent cancer-fighting nutrients. They are also major helper foods for the liver and the processing of toxins, which is a must for any weight-loss quest.

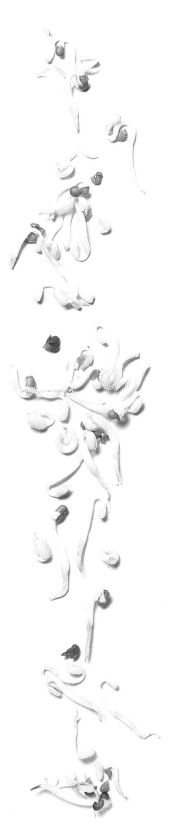

Day 18

BREAKFAST

1 cup of warm water
1 cup of Lemongrass tea
followed by a bowl of stewed prunes with
one ripe chopped pear, and a bowl of Oat
Groat Porridge.

Oat Groat Porridge
SERVES 1
125g oat groats
400ml rice milk or water – rice milk for
extra sweetness

1. Put the oat groats and water or rice milk
in a pot and bring to the boil. Lower the
heat and simmer until the groats thicken.
2. Turn off the heat and allow the porridge
to sit for a few minutes.
3. Sprinkle with cinnamon and serve.

MID-MORNING SNACK
One apple and one pear.

LUNCH

Miso soup (from packet) followed by vegetable crudités with Cashew and Brazil Nut Paté.

Cashew and Brazil Nut Paté

This mixture will keep well in the fridge for up to two days.

SERVES 4
100g plain Brazil nuts, roughly chopped
100g plain cashew nuts, roughly chopped
2 tsp olive oil
1 garlic clove, peeled and roughly chopped
1 tbsp freshly squeezed lemon juice
small bunch fresh parsley
4 tbsp cold water

1. Whiz all the ingredients together in a food processor until almost smooth – you may need to remove the lid and push the mixture down a few times until the right consistency is reached.
2. Serve with lots of fresh vegetable crudités of your choice.

MID-AFTERNOON SNACK

Veggie Juice or four baby gem lettuce leaves with houmous, cherry tomatoes, grated carrot and dill.

Veggie Juice

SERVES 1
3 broccoli florets
6 carrots
2 celery stalks
4 tomatoes

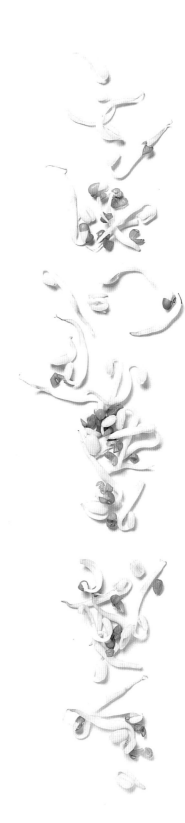

DINNER

Cinnamon Chicken with Minted Salad or Lentil
and Vegetable 'Lasagne' with side salad.

Cinnamon Chicken with Minted Salad

SERVES 2

2 small boneless, skinless chicken breasts
(total weight around 250g)
1/2 tsp ground cinnamon
1/2 tsp ground cumin
2 tbsp chopped fresh coriander
1 garlic clove, peeled and crushed
freshly squeezed juice of half a lemon
1 tsp virgin olive oil
lemon wedges, to serve

FOR THE SALAD

4 heaped tbsp frozen peas
2 spring onions, trimmed
and diagonally sliced
3 ripe vine tomatoes, roughly chopped
75g cucumber, cut into 1cm dice
2 tbsp roughly chopped fresh mint leaves
1 little gem lettuce, leaves separated,
washed and drained

1. Cut each chicken breast into eight
chunks and place in a non-metallic bowl.
Add the cinnamon, cumin, coriander, garlic,
lemon juice and olive oil. Cover and chill
for 30 minutes.

2. Preheat the oven to 200C/Gas 6. Line
a large baking tray with non-stick foil.

3. Lift the chicken out of the marinade
using a fork and shake off any excess.
Place the pieces on the foil-lined tray,
spaced well apart.

4. Bake for around 15–18 minutes until
the chicken is cooked through.

5. Cook the peas in boiling water for
2 minutes. Drain in a sieve then plunge
into a bowl of cold water to cool.

6. Drain the peas once more and toss with
the spring onions, tomatoes, cucumber
and mint.

7. Divide the lettuce leaves between two
plates and top with the minted salad.

8. Serve the hot chicken with the salad
and lemon wedges for squeezing.

My Mum used to tell me that I had to eat my porridge
oats cause they would 'stick tae my ribs and keep me
warm'. What Mum did not know is that oats can do a
lot more than keep my insides warm. You can sow your
wild oats, literally. Oats have been found to increase
sexual desire.

Lentil and Vegetable 'Lasagne'

This recipe can be prepared ahead. Simply follow all the steps then allow to cool. Cover and chill until required. It will keep for up to 24 hours. Cook from the fridge for 10–15 minutes until hot throughout.

SERVES 2

1 tbsp olive oil
1 medium onion, peeled and chopped
2 garlic cloves, peeled and crushed
1 yellow pepper, de-seeded and cut into 1cm dice
1 medium courgette, trimmed and cut into 1cm dice
75g red split lentils, rinsed
227-g can chopped tomatoes
700ml just-boiled water
2 tsp organic vegetable bouillon powder
1 large leek, trimmed to a length of 14cm
30g plain mixed nuts, chopped (optional)

1. Heat the oil in a large saucepan and gently water-fry the onion, garlic, pepper and courgette for 10 minutes until softened but not coloured, stirring regularly.
2. Add the lentils and turn to coat in the oil.
3. Stir in the tomatoes, water and bouillon powder. Bring to the boil, then reduce the heat slightly and simmer for about 25 minutes or until the lentils are tender and the liquid is reduced and thickened. Stir regularly, especially towards the end of the cooking time.
4. While the lentils are cooking, bring a large pan of water to the boil. Cut the leek in half lengthways and separate the layers. Add the leek to the boiling water and cook for 5 minutes or until very tender.
5. Preheat the oven to 200C/Gas 6.
6. Drain the leek in a colander and cool under cold running water.
7. Remove the lentil mixture from the heat and spoon a third into the base of a 1.5 ltr rectangular ovenproof dish. Arrange half the sliced leek over the lentils. Top with another third of the lentils and the remaining leek. Finish with the rest of the lentil mixture and sprinkle with the nuts if using.
8. Bake for 15 minutes until hot.
9. Serve with a lightly dressed mixed salad.

Day 19

BREAKFAST

1 cup of warm water
followed by Avocado and Lime Shake.

Avocado and Lime Shake
SERVES 2
1 ripe avocado, halved and stoned
freshly squeezed juice of 1 lime
3 fresh dates, skinned and stoned (or figs)
450ml cold water

1. Using a dessertspoon, scoop the avocado flesh into a food processor or liquidizer.
2. Add the lime juice, dates and water.
3. Blend until smooth and serve in tall glasses.

MID-MORNING SNACK
Bowl of fresh pineapple chunks or one plum and one peach.

LUNCH
Hearty Miso Soup with brown rice and spinach, followed by vegetable crudités and cashew dip.

Hearty Miso Soup
Simply make up a bowl of miso soup from the packet and add some cooked brown rice and fresh, raw spinach leaves.

Creamy Cashew Dip
This recipe makes enough to serve four, so save some for snacking on with crudités tomorrow.

2 tbsp cashew nut butter
2 tbsp just-boiled water
few drops Tamari sauce

1. Blend the cashew nut butter with 2 tsp of the just-boiled water in a small bowl until smooth.
2. Gradually add the remaining water, stirring well between each addition.
3. Season with a few drops of Tamari sauce and stir until creamy.
4. Serve with vegetable crudités of your choice.

MID-AFTERNOON SNACK
Handful of unsalted mixed nuts or seeds.

DINNER
Herb Baked Cod with Oven Roasted Vegetables.

Tomato and Herb Baked Cod
Save some veggies for tomorrow's lunch.

SERVES 2
2 150g fresh, skinless cod fillets
2 vine-ripened tomatoes, sliced
1 good pinch dried mixed herbs

1. Preheat the oven to 200C/Gas 6. Place the fillets of cod on to two squares of foil – each roughly 4cm larger than the fish itself. Bring the sides up slightly to create a shallow foil bowl. Place on a baking tray.
2. Top each fillet with three slices of tomato and season with a pinch of dried herbs.
3. Bake for about 12 minutes until the fish is cooked – it should look opaque and flake easily.
4. Lift carefully on to two warmed plates, slide off the foil and drizzle with the cooking juices to serve.

Simple Roasted Vegetables
SERVES 3–4
2 medium courgettes, trimmed and cut into 1cm slices
1 red pepper, de-seeded and cut into 2.5cm pieces
1 yellow pepper, de-seeded and cut into 2.5cm pieces
8 shallots, peeled and halved (quartered if large)
2 tbsp olive oil

1. Preheat the oven to 200C/Gas 6.
2. Place the courgettes, peppers and shallots on a large baking tray. Drizzle with the oil and toss together lightly.
3. Bake for 35 minutes until tender and lightly browned, carefully turning halfway through the cooking time. Serve piping hot.

SOAK YOUR BARLEY OVERNIGHT READY FOR MAKING BREAKFAST SOUP.

If you want something sweet, opt for a piece of fruit or a root vegetable. They taste naturally sweet and should satisfy any sweet desires. And the more you chew your foods, the sweeter they taste.

Day 20

BREAKFAST

1 cup of warm water
1 cup of Nettle tea
followed by melon slices and Breakfast Barley Soup.
Remember to wait 20 minutes between eating the fruit and the soup.

Breakfast Barley Soup
Soak the barley overnight, otherwise you will have to call in late for work! When you soak a grain like barley, it makes the cooking more rapid.

SERVES 1
4 tbsps pearl barley
2 sachets white miso
4 shitake mushrooms

1. Drain the barley.
2. Bring 125ml water to the boil and add the barley.
3. Bring back to the boil, lower the heat and simmer for 10 minutes.
4. Add the white miso and shitake mushrooms, simmer for a further five minutes and then serve.

MID-MORNING SNACK
Two pears.

LUNCH
Oven Roasted Veggies from yesterday, with rocket leaves and cous cous.

Oven Roasted Veggies
SERVES 1
reserved portion of oven roasted vegetables
1 tbsp cider vinegar
2 tbsp pine nuts
a handful of rocket leaves
olive oil

1. Toss the oven roasted vegetables with the cider vinegar, pine nuts and rocket leaves.
2. Drizzle with a little extra olive oil to serve.
3. Serve with a small bowl of plain cous cous if you feel extra hungry.

MID-AFTERNOON SNACK
Creamy Cashew Dip (see Day 19) with vegetable crudités.

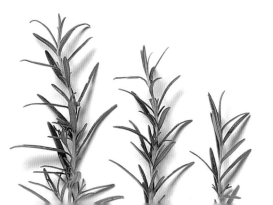
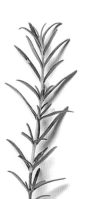
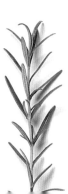
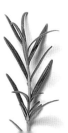

DINNER
Bean Cassoulet with brown rice.

Bean Cassoulet
SERVES 2
1 onion, finely chopped
1 leek, washed and cut into 1 cm pieces
2 cloves garlic
1 tsp olive oil
2 tbsp water
1 300-g can no salt, no sugar
Flageolet beans, drained
1 200-g can no salt, no sugar
Borlotti beans, drained
2 sprigs of rosemary
1 tsp fennel seeds
few sprigs of thyme
1 tbsp millet flour
3 tomatoes, de-seeded and finely chopped
2 tbsp parsley

1. Place the onion, leek, garlic, oil and water in a non-stick pan and cover and cook for 4–5 minutes until soft.
2. Transfer to an earthenware dish and mix in the beans. Scatter with the herbs (except parsley) and half the tomatoes.
3. Preheat the oven to 180C/Gas 4.
4. Bake the cassoulet for 10 minutes. Remove from the oven and give the mixture a stir. Then sprinkle on the millet flour. Return to the oven and bake for a further 10 minutes.
5. Sprinkle over the remaining tomatoes and parsley and serve with brown rice or a green salad.

When eating fruit, keep your melons separate from your other fruits. Melon digests faster than all other fruits. If you mix them with other fruits, you will be fermenting away in your gut and you know what that means ...GAS!

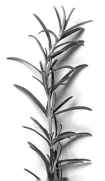
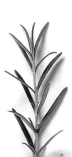
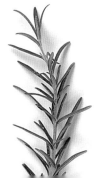

Day 21

BREAKFAST

1 cup of warm water
1 cup of Sage tea
followed by a smoothie.

Berry, Mango and Banana Smoothie
In the winter, you could always warm up the
fruit for a change – but if you want to pour
your warm smoothies over fruit, make sure
the fruit is raw.

SERVES 1
1 tub raspberries
1 mango, stoned and chopped
1 banana

Blend until smooth.

MID-MORNING SNACK
Bowl of grapes.

LUNCH
Fennel, Cauliflower and Celery Salad.

Fennel, Cauliflower and Celery Salad
Fresh miso paste is available at the chilled
counter at health food shops and is a good
base for salad dressings as well as soups
and stews.

SERVES 4
320g fresh cauliflower florets
200g celery, sliced
200g fennel bulb, cored and chopped
4 tsp shelled hemp seeds
FOR THE DRESSING
2 tsp fresh miso paste with hemp
2 tbsp mirin
juice of 1 lemon

1. Steam the cauliflower florets for 3 minutes
until just tender.
2. Mix in a bowl with the celery and fennel.
3. In a small jar, mix the miso paste, mirin
and lemon juice. Mix or shake well.
4. Pour the dressing over the salad, sprinkle
with the seeds and serve.

MID-AFTERNOON SNACK
Veggie Juice or a handful of salt-free organic almonds
(if you can soak the almonds first in water they will be
even easier to digest).

Veggie Juice
SERVES 1
1 cucumber
6 carrots
1 fennel
1/2 beetroot

DINNER

Speedy Sweet Potato Soup and Shitake Mushroom and Green Bean Salad with Sesame and Spring Onion Dressing.

Speedy Sweet Potato Soup

Save some for lunch tomorrow. If you don't have a stick blender, allow the soup to cool before blending in a food processor or liquidizer until smooth. Return to the pan and heat through gently.

SERVES 4

1 medium onion, peeled and roughly chopped
1 garlic clove, peeled and crushed
2 sweet potatoes, peeled and cut into 2cm chunks
2 medium carrots, peeled and thinly sliced
800ml just-boiled water
½ vegetable stock cube

1. Put all the ingredients in a saucepan and bring to the boil. Simmer for about 15 minutes until the vegetables are very tender.
2. Remove from the heat. Cool for a few minutes, then blend using a stick blender until smooth.
3. Add some extra water if necessary and warm through gently to serve.

Shitake Mushroom and Green Bean Salad with Sesame and Spring Onion Dressing

Furikake – a combination of black and white sesame seeds, nori seaweed and red shiso leaves – is available from health food shops and oriental groceries. If you can't find it then use sesame seeds.

SERVES 2

75g green beans, ends trimmed
60g mushrooms, preferably shitake, stalks removed and finely sliced
1 tbsp furikake seasoning
FOR THE DRESSING
2 spring onions, white part only
1 tsp sesame oil
1 tbsp brown rice vinegar

1. Bring a small pan of water to the boil, add the beans and cook for 1 minute. Drain and rinse well under cold running water.
2. In a small bowl mix the spring onions, oil and vinegar.
3. Arrange the beans on a serving plate and top with the sliced mushrooms. Spoon over the dressing then scatter with furikake and serve.

REMEMBER TO SOAK YOUR BLACK TURTLE BEANS FOR TOMORROW – 100G IN PLENTY OF COLD WATER OVERNIGHT.

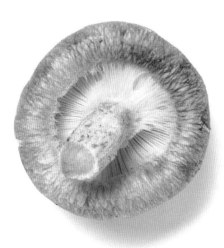

Day 22

BREAKFAST

1 cup of warm water
1 cup Lemon Balm tea
followed by a fruit salad of seasonal fruits,
and if you are still hungry, a bowl of porridge.
Pop a cup of chickpeas into water and soak
until tomorrow (this is for a snack).

Fruit Salad
Stewed apples and prunes served in
a warmed breakfast bowl, garnished
with a pinch of cinnamon.

Quick Porridge Oats with Cinnamon and Vanilla
SERVES 1
100g porridge oats
400ml water
2cm stick of cinnamon
vanilla pod, split in half lengthways

1. Place the oats and water in a small
saucepan and place over a moderate to high
heat, stir well then add the cinnamon and
vanilla pod.
2. Bring to the boil without stirring. Simmer
for 1 minute while stirring, until the mixture
becomes thick and creamy.
3. Remove from the heat when it reaches
your preferred consistency. Pour into a bowl
and discard the vanilla and cinnamon.
Serve immediately.

MID-MORNING SNACK
One tub of blueberries.

LUNCH
Speedy Sweet Potato Soup with salad.

Carrot and Pea Salad with Fresh Ginger
SERVES 1
125g carrot, peeled
60g shelled fresh peas
freshly grated ginger, to taste
1/2 tbsp brown rice vinegar

1. Slice the carrot very finely, if possible
with a mandolin, and then place in a bowl
with the peas.
2. Grate some fresh ginger to taste,
add it to the peas and carrot.
3. Pour over the vinegar and serve.

MID-AFTERNOON SNACK
Handful of raw sugar snap peas or mangetout
and a handful of pumpkin seeds.

**Vegetable Rissoles with raw mangetout and
Sweet Corn Relish.**

Vegetable Rissoles

Use a good quality non-stick pan and there
is no need to use any more than a slight
wipe of oil over the surface before cooking
the rissoles.

SERVES 4
100g Black Turtle beans
10g arame seaweed
1 medium onion, finely chopped
1 tsp oil and 1 tbsp water
1/2 yellow pepper, finely diced
100g peeled, grated swede
100g courgette, grated
2 tbsp chopped parsley
1 clove garlic, peeled and finely chopped
100g millet flour
a little oil to grease

1. Soak the beans in a bowl of cold water
overnight. Drain them and put them in
a pan of cold water. Bring to the boil and
simmer for 45 minutes. Drain and mash
with a potato masher.
2. Soak the arame in cold water for
10 minutes and drain.
3. Place the onion in a non-stick pan with
1 tsp of oil and 1 tbsp of cold water, water-fry
gently to soften but do not brown.

4. Mix the cooked beans, arame, pepper,
swede, courgette, parsley and garlic and
stir well. Then mix in the millet flour.
5. Form into 8 round balls.
6. Preheat a non-stick pan and take
a little oil on a pastry brush and lightly oil
the surface of the pan. Place 4 balls in the
pan and with a flat spatula press down to
flatten. Cook for 2–3 minutes until golden
in colour. Turn the rissoles over and cook
for a further 2–3 minutes until golden in
colour. Remove from the pan and repeat
with the other rissoles.
7. Serve with raw mangetout, a squeeze
of lemon juice and Sweet Corn Relish.

Sweet Corn Relish
This will keep for 1–2 days in the fridge.

SERVES 4
150-g can organic tinned sweet corn
1/2 red pepper, finely diced
1/2 red onion, finely diced
2 tsp cider vinegar

1. Mix all the ingredients together and
place in a clean jar until required.

Go for shitakes. These mushrooms have been found
to have powerful, immune-enhancing properties. I want
my clients to develop strong immune systems so it's a
good veggie to toss into salads, soups and stews. Other
interesting varieties are reishi, maitake and enochi.

Day 23

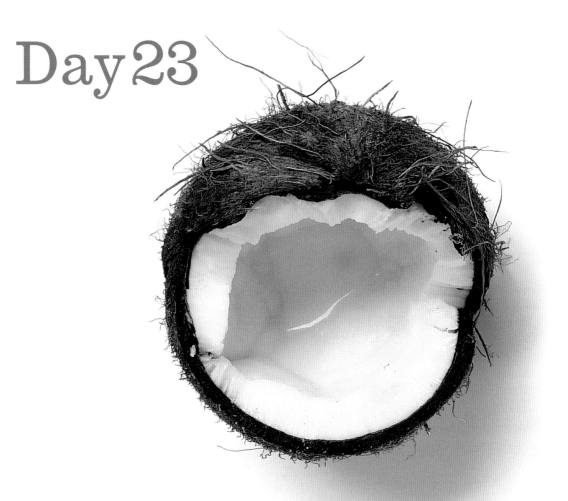

BREAKFAST

1 cup of **warm water**
1 cup of **Dandelion tea**
followed by a smoothie.

Peach, Apricot and Banana Smoothie
SERVES 1
2 ripe peaches, halved and stoned
4 apricots
1 banana
100ml water

Blend until smooth.

MID-MORNING SNACK
Bowl of sprouted mung beans sprinkled with
sesame seeds and a squeeze of lemon.

LUNCH
Avocado Stuffed with Black Eye Peas.

Avocado Stuffed with Black Eye Peas
Share this one with friends. They will
love this dish.

SERVES 2
**1 avocado, halved, stone removed
squeeze of lemon juice
300-g can of Black Eye Peas, drained.
(You will only use half of the can here,
save the rest for tomorrow)
100g cherry tomatoes, halved
1 spring onion, chopped
1/2 tbsp cider vinegar
1 tbsp fresh basil**

1. Place the avocado halves on serving
plates and sprinkle over the lemon juice.
2. Mix all the other ingredients together
and spoon into the avocados.
3. Serve immediately.

MID-AFTERNOON SNACK
**Remember the chickpeas you soaked overnight?
They should now be just starting to sprout and so will
be packed with food enzymes. Drain and serve.**

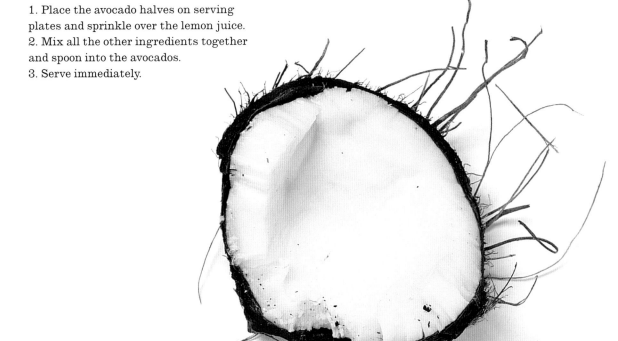

DINNER
Vegetable juice made from carrot, cucumber and celery, followed by Asparagus Risotto.

Asparagus Risotto
Reserve a portion for tomorrow's lunch.

SERVES 4
1 bunch fresh asparagus
1 leek, halved and thinly sliced,
reserve the trimmings
1 ltr water
1 bay leaf
2 cloves garlic
1 tsp olive oil
2 tbsp water (for water frying)
300g short grain brown rice
2 tbsp flat leaf parsley
1 tbsp lemon juice
handful fresh rocket

1. Take the asparagus spears and snap the tough base from the stem. The asparagus will naturally break at the best point. Chop the asparagus into 1.5cm pieces.
2. Place the leek trimmings and the discarded asparagus bases in a medium sized pan, pour in the water and bring to the boil. Add the bay leaf and leave to simmer.
3. In a non-stick frying pan heat the oil with 2 tbsp water and add the sliced leek and garlic. Cook for 5 minutes to soften but not colour, then spoon in 2 tbsp of the asparagus water from the simmering pan.
4. Add the rice and cook for a few minutes stirring continuously. Then add 200ml of the simmering asparagus water, cook for a few minutes until the rice absorbs all the water and then add a further 200ml of asparagus water.

5. Continue to add the hot asparagus liquid to the rice and cook over a gentle heat for approximately 30 minutes. The rice should require about 800ml of liquid. Discard the leek and asparagus trimmings.
6. Add the chopped asparagus to the rice, stir well and simmer for a further 5 minutes. Add the parsley and lemon juice. If required, add a little more stock. The rice should be tender and moist.
7. Serve the risotto in warmed soup plates and scatter with the fresh rocket.

If you want to lose weight, eat raw shelled hemp seeds. I call it my Weight Loss Seed. Raw shelled hemp contains the perfect ratio of the good fats which will help to burn fat in your body. It has a fabulous mineral profile and a good source of the much needed, sex-boosting nutrient, zinc. Use raw shelled hemp seeds liberally as a snack, in soups, stews and dips.

Day 24

BREAKFAST

1 cup of warm water with a squeeze of lemon
1 cup of Sage tea
followed by a Peach and Mango Smoothie.

Peach and Mango Smoothie
SERVES 1
1 mango, stoned and chopped
1 peach, stoned and chopped
1 banana, sliced
100ml water
1 small tub blueberries

1. Blend all ingredients (except blueberries) until smooth.
2. Add more water if you want a thinner consistency.
3. Pour over the blueberries and drink.

MID-MORNING SNACK
Juice of a pink grapefruit and two apples or grapefruit segments.

LUNCH
Asparagus Risotto from yesterday, with Southern Style Black Eye Pea Salad.

Southern Style Black Eye Pea Salad with Red Onions and Peppers
Remember the black eye peas you had left over yesterday? Here's where you use them. This salad will keep well in the fridge for three days.

remainder of 300-g can
of Black Eye Peas, drained.
1/2 red onion, finely chopped
1/2 red pepper, cored, de-seeded
and finely chopped
1/2 yellow pepper, cored, de-seeded
and finely chopped
FOR THE DRESSING
1 tbsp fresh coriander, chopped
1/2 tsp Dijon mustard
1/2 tbsp cider vinegar
1/2 tbsp olive oil

1. Mix the beans, onion and peppers together.
2. Place the dressing ingredients in a jar and shake well.
3. Pour the dressing over the beans, stir well, cover and chill.
4. Leave to marinade for 2–3 hours before serving for extra flavour, or simply eat straightaway.

MID-AFTERNOON SNACK
Veggie Juice or a red or yellow pepper, sliced.

Veggie Juice
SERVES 1
1 fennel
1/2 beetroot
4 celery stalks

DINNER
Salmon and Savoy Cabbage 'Lasagne'.

Salmon and Savoy Cabbage 'Lasagne'

This dish gets its name from the layers of cabbage and salmon that resemble a traditional lasagne. It is full of flavour and is really good for entertaining.

SERVES 4
1 large savoy cabbage
2 tsp sesame oil
3 tbsp boiling water
zest of 1 lemon
2 tsp brown rice vinegar
1 tsp wheat-free soy sauce
300g fillet of salmon
8 spring onions, finely chopped

1. Remove the outer leaves from the cabbage and discard. Take 5 leaves from the cabbage and remove the tough central vein. This will leave a small 'V' shape in the leaf.
2. Bring a large pan of water to the boil and add the 5 leaves. Boil for 2 minutes. Drain and refresh in cold water.
3. Finely shred the remaining cabbage and place in a non-stick pan with the sesame oil and boiling water. Place on a moderate heat and cook until the cabbage has just wilted, than add the lemon zest, rice vinegar and soy sauce. Remove from the heat and leave in the pan to cool.

4. Place the salmon fillet on a chopping board and with a sharp knife slice the fish horizontally into $1/2$ cm slices.
5. Take a large piece of greaseproof paper and place a cabbage leaf in the centre. Cover with half of the salmon slices. With a slotted spoon place half of the shredded cabbage mixture on top. Cover with a second cabbage leaf and repeat the process until you have completed the lasagne.
6. Drizzle a little of the cooking juice from the shredded cabbage over the top. Wrap the paper firmly around the salmon and cabbage.
7. Place the parcel in a bamboo steamer over a pan of boiling water and steam for 7–10 minutes. The parcel will feel firm to the touch.
8. Remove from the steamer, unwrap and slice into 4 wedges. Transfer to 4 warm serving plates and drizzle over any remaining juices.
9. Scatter the chopped spring onions over the top and serve immediately.

Day 25

BREAKFAST

1 cup of warm water
1 cup of Nettle and Dandelion tea combined
followed by Quinoa Vanilla Porridge

Quinoa Vanilla Porridge
SERVES 2
150g quinoa grains
1/2 vanilla pod
350ml water or rice milk

1. Combine the quinoa, vanilla pod and
water or rice milk in a pan.
2. Bring to the boil, then lower the heat
and simmer for approx 10 minutes, or
until the grains are translucent.
3. Take off the heat and allow to stand
for a few minutes before serving.

MID-MORNING SNACK
Two fresh figs, or dried (unsulphured) if you can't get fresh.

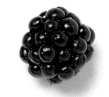

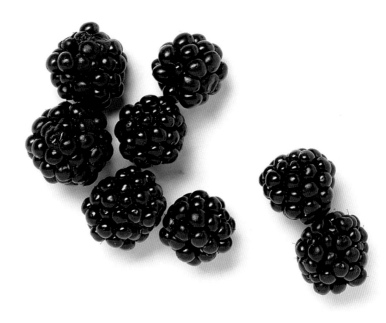

LUNCH
Watercress Soup with Turnip, and Avocado,
Tomato and Basil Salad.

Watercress Soup with Turnip

This soup has a fantastic peppery taste
and is best made whilst organic watercress
is in season through the summer months.
It should be made when the watercress is
very fresh, and cooked and eaten on the
same day to preserve its nutritional value.
If watercress is unavailable then replace
with lettuce leaves.

SERVES 2
1 bunch (125g) watercress (or lettuce)
1 onion, finely chopped
1 tsp olive oil
2 tbsp water
100g white turnips, peeled and chopped
750ml home-made stock or water

1. Trim the leaves from $1/2$ bunch of
the watercress (if using) and set aside
for garnish.
2. Place the onion, oil and water in
a medium-sized pan, cover and cook
until soft but not coloured.
3. Add the turnips and stock, bring to
the boil and simmer for 20–30 minutes
until the turnips are soft when pierced
with a knife.
4. Add the watercress (or lettuce) and
cook for barely 1 minute, remove from
the heat and allow to cool slightly.
5. Pour the soup into the processor or
blender and blend until smooth.
6. Serve in four warmed serving
bowls and garnish with the reserved
watercress leaves.

Avocado, Tomato and Basil Salad
SERVES 2
2 ripe avocados, halved
4 medium vine-ripened tomatoes, sliced
2 handfuls fresh basil leaves
15g pine nuts
2 tbsp extra virgin olive oil
1 tsp good quality balsamic vinegar

1. Stone the avocados and slice thickly.
Peel off the skin and discard.
2. Arrange the avocado slices on two
serving plates and top with the tomatoes
and basil leaves. Sprinkle with the pine nuts.
3. Drizzle with olive oil and balsamic vinegar
to serve.

MID-AFTERNOON SNACK
Tub of blueberries or raspberries.

DINNER
Chinese Cabbage Casserole.

Chinese Cabbage Casserole
Reserve a portion for lunch tomorrow.

SERVES 4
1 ltr water
2cm piece fresh ginger, sliced
1 tsp coriander seeds, crushed
1 clove garlic, peeled
600g Chinese cabbage
100g Daikon (or radish), peeled
and cut into julienne or matchsticks
100g carrots, peeled and sliced
4 tbsp fresh coriander, chopped
1 tsp sesame oil
1 tsp wheat-free soy sauce
1 tbsp sesame seeds
20g arame soaked in cold water
for 10 minutes and drained

1. Place the water, ginger, coriander seeds and garlic in a medium to large saucepan. Bring to the boil.

2. Add the cabbage, Daikon and carrot and simmer for 5 minutes.

3. Remove from the heat and stir in half the coriander.

4. Spoon into soup bowls and drizzle over the oil, soy sauce, sesame seeds, remaining coriander and arame. Serve.

SOAK 80G ADZUKI BEANS IN PLENTY OF COLD WATER OVERNIGHT READY FOR TOMORROW.

Day 26

BREAKFAST

1 cup of warm water
1 cup of Spearmint or Fennel tea
followed by a smoothie.

Strawberry Smoothie
SERVES 1
1 small punnet strawberries, hulled
1/2 tub raspberries
2 ripe pears, cored and chopped
1 apple, peeled and chopped
200ml water

Blend all the ingredients until smooth.

MID-MORNING SNACK
Houmous with a selection of seeds:
pumpkin, sunflower or raw shelled hemp.

LUNCH
Chinese Cabbage Casserole from yesterday, served with a steamed corn on the cob that you have rubbed with umeboshi plum sauce.

MID-AFTERNOON SNACK
Half a cucumber, finely chopped.

DINNER
Adzuki Bean Mini Burgers with Onion Gravy.

Reserve a portion of Burgers and Onion Gravy for tomorrow.

Always, always opt for brown rice over white if you want to have energy and stay slim. White rice is stripped of too many nutrients and tends to behave like sugar in the body. Brown rice is a good source of B vitamins which are critical for adrenal function and weight balance. Recent research has found that eating a diet rich in whole grains such as brown rice can help to control weight gain. So now you know…

Adzuki Bean Mini Burgers

If you boil the soaked adzuki beans for about 40 minutes until very soft, they will blend better in the food processor.

MAKES 12 BURGERS
75g mixed unsalted nuts, roughly chopped (I use pine nuts)
180g soft cooked adzuki beans
2 tbsp Tahini (sesame paste)
50g roughly chopped onion
2 tbsp chopped fresh parsley
1 tsp organic vegetable bouillon powder
1 tsp olive oil

1. Preheat the oven to 200C/Gas 6. Cover a baking tray with non-stick foil.
2. Place the nuts in a food processor and blend until finely ground. Add the adzuki beans, Tahini, onion, parsley and stock.
3. Blend until the mixture forms an almost smooth, thick paste – you may have to remove the lid and push the mixture down once or twice until the right consistency is reached. Roll into 12 small balls with clean hands and place on the baking tray. Flatten into small burger shapes.
4. Brush the burgers lightly with the oil and bake for 10 minutes. Remove from the oven and carefully turn over using a spatula. Return to the oven for a further 5–7 minutes until the burgers are cooked through and lightly browned.
5. Serve the burgers with Onion gravy or Zesty Avocado 'mayo' (page 98), plus a large mixed salad or lots of seasonal vegetables.

Onion Gravy

3 onions
3 tbsp olive oil
2 tsp Tamari sauce

1. Sweat the onions in the olive oil on a low heat for 15 minutes until soft and translucent. You are not frying them.
2. Add a little water under the onions and cook them for another 10–15 minutes.
3. Blend the onions and pour into a bowl. Add the Tamari sauce and serve.

Day 27

BREAKFAST

1 cup of warm water
1 cup of Nettle tea

Fruit Smoothie
It's got to be a smoothie and one that
you concoct. So get busy. And let me
know what you come up with.

MID-MORNING SNACK
One tub of blueberries.

LUNCH
Left-over Adzuki Bean Burgers with Onion Gravy
from yesterday.

MID-AFTERNOON SNACK
Bowl of raw sauerkraut (rinsed).

DINNER
Minced Turkey Meatballs with Surprise Tomato Sauce
and crunchy salad, or Chickpea Vegetable Stew.

**Minced Turkey Meatballs with
Surprise Tomato Sauce**
The sauce is optional and the meatballs
are equally delicious simply served with
a leafy green salad and a squeeze of lemon.

SERVES 4
**500g fresh turkey mince, preferably organic
or free range
1 medium onion, peeled and finely chopped
1 garlic clove, peeled and crushed
1 small bunch fresh coriander, finely chopped
1/2 tsp organic wheat-free vegetable bouillon
powder**
FOR THE SAUCE
**400-g can chopped tomatoes
1 garlic clove, peeled and chopped
1 medium onion, peeled and roughly chopped
1 celery stick, trimmed and thinly sliced
1 large carrot, peeled and thinly sliced
1 sweet potato, peeled and cubed
1 leek, trimmed and finely sliced
1 courgette, trimmed and cubed
1 bay leaf (optional)**

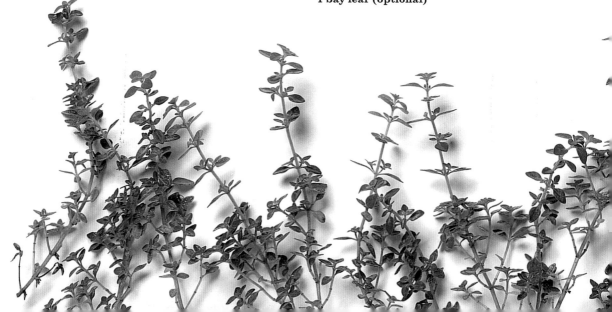

1. Place all the sauce ingredients in a large saucepan. Fill the empty tomato can with cold water and pour over the vegetables. Bring to the boil, then reduce the heat and simmer gently for 25–30 minutes until the vegetables are tender and the sauce is thick, stirring regularly.

2. Meanwhile, preheat the oven to 200C/ Gas 6. Place the turkey mince in a large bowl and, using clean hands, mix thoroughly with the onion, garlic, coriander and bouillon powder.

3. Form the mince mixture into 20 small balls and place on a baking tray lined with foil. Bake for 12–15 minutes, turning halfway through the cooking time, until the turkey is lightly browned and cooked through.

4. Allow the cooked sauce to cool for 5 minutes. Discard the bay leaf, if using, and then carefully blend the sauce until smooth.

5. Return to the pan and stir in the meatballs. Heat through gently together until the sauce is hot.

6. Serve with a crisp, crunchy raw salad.

VEGETARIAN ALTERNATIVE
Chickpea Vegetable Stew
SERVES 2

1 red onion, sliced
2 garlic cloves, crushed
1 tbsp hemp oil or olive oil
1 red pepper, diced
1 courgette, sliced
1 leek, sliced
1 400-g can of no salt, no sugar, chickpeas
625ml/1.2 cups cold water
2 tsp wheat-free vegetable bouillon stock powder
handful baby spinach leaves

1. Sweat the onion and garlic in the oil over a low heat until the onion is soft.

2. Stir in the red pepper, courgette and leek. Rinse the chickpeas and add them to the onion and pepper mixture.

3. Add the water and bouillon powder and bring to the boil. Reduce the heat and simmer for 6–8 minutes until the vegetables are just tender.

4. Stir in the baby spinach leaves at the last moment and serve with freshly cooked brown rice.

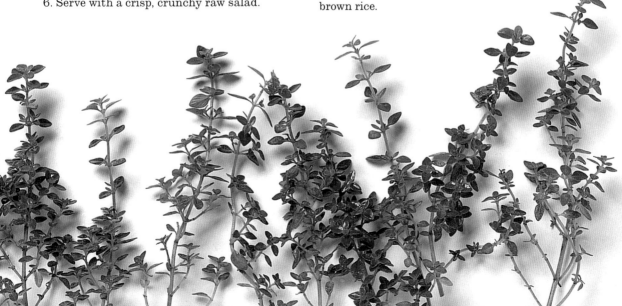

Day 28

BREAKFAST

1 cup of warm water
1 cup of Nettle tea
followed by Warm Fruit.

Warm Fruit
1 apple
1 pear
2 peaches
2 apricots
Chop all the fruit and warm through in
a pan with 100ml of pressed apple juice
before serving.

MID-MORNING SNACK
Two grated carrots and one grated beetroot with a handful
of alfalfa sprouts and a squeeze of lemon.

LUNCH

**Chilled Fennel Soup with Avocado
and Cucumber**
SERVES 2
1 tsp olive oil
**2 fennel bulbs, chopped, with the tough
core removed**
½ Daikon (or radish), peeled and chopped
1 bay leaf
1 tsp coriander seeds
250ml vegetable stock
½ cucumber, finely diced
1 avocado, finely diced
juice of ½ lemon

1. Heat the oil in a non-stick pan, add a little
water, and sweat the fennel for 2 minutes.
2. Add the Daikon, bay leaf, coriander seeds
and vegetable stock and simmer until the
fennel is tender – 20–25 minutes.
3. Pass the mixture through a Mouli
or coarse sieve. Allow to cool.
4. Mix the cucumber with the avocado and
the lemon juice. Mix into the soup and chill
before serving.

Do not eat standing up or when running
around on the go. Sit down when you are
eating a meal or a snack. You will digest
your food far more effectively when you
are relaxed.

Broccoli Salad with Pine Nuts

SERVES 2
1 head broccoli, cut into florets
1/2 red onion, diced
10 cherry tomatoes, halved
2 tbsp basil, chopped
2 tbsp pine nuts, lightly toasted
1 tbsp tamarind
juice of half a lemon

1. Bring a pan of water to the boil and blanch the broccoli for 1 minute.
2. Strain in a colander and run under cold water. Allow to drain. This prevents the broccoli from losing its colour and nutrients.
3. Place the broccoli in a salad bowl with the onion, tomato and basil.
4. Mix the pine nuts with the tamarind and lemon juice and spoon over the salad.

MID-AFTERNOON SNACK
Cucumber and carrot crudités with houmous, sprinkled with dill.

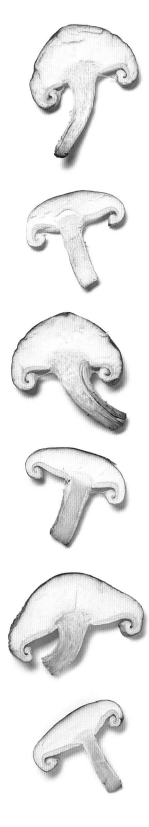

DINNER
Bean Bangers with Onion Gravy and freshly cooked vegetables.

Bean Bangers with Onion Gravy

If you are making this dish to serve 3, make 6 fat sausages instead of 8 thinner ones and cook for 1–2 minutes longer.

SERVES 3–4

100g shelled mixed nuts such as Brazil, hazelnut, almonds, walnuts and pecans, roughly chopped
50g onion, roughly chopped
1 clove garlic, peeled and halved
300-g can red kidney beans, drained and rinsed under cold water in a colander
2 tbsp roughly chopped fresh parsley
1 tsp organic vegetable bouillon powder
1 tsp virgin olive oil
FOR THE ONION GRAVY
1 tsp virgin olive oil
50g onion, thinly sliced
175ml just-boiled water
2 tsp organic wheat-free Tamari sauce
1 1/2–2 tsp ground arrowroot blended with 2–3 tsp cold water

1. Preheat the oven to 200C/Gas 6. Line a baking sheet with non-stick foil.
2. Place the nuts in a food processor and blend until very finely chopped.
3. Add the onion, garlic, kidney beans, parsley and bouillon powder. Blend until the mixture forms an almost smooth, thick paste – you may have to push the mixture down with a spatula once or twice until the right consistency is reached.
4. Form the mixture into 8 balls with clean hands, then roll into sausage shapes (about 9cm long) and place on the baking tray.

5. Brush the sausages all over with a little oil and bake for 10 minutes. Carefully remove the tray from the oven and turn the sausages over. Cook for a further 5–7 minutes until lightly browned and hot throughout.
6. While the sausages are cooking, prepare the gravy. Place the oil and onion in a small saucepan with 1 tbsp cold water and cook over a low heat for about 5 minutes until the onion is softened and very lightly browned, stirring regularly.
7. Add the just-boiled water and Tamari sauce and bring to the boil. Stir in the arrowroot mixture – less arrowroot will make a thinner gravy – and cook for 1 minute, stirring constantly until the sauce is thickened and glossy.
8. Serve the sausages with the gravy and lots of freshly cooked vegetables.

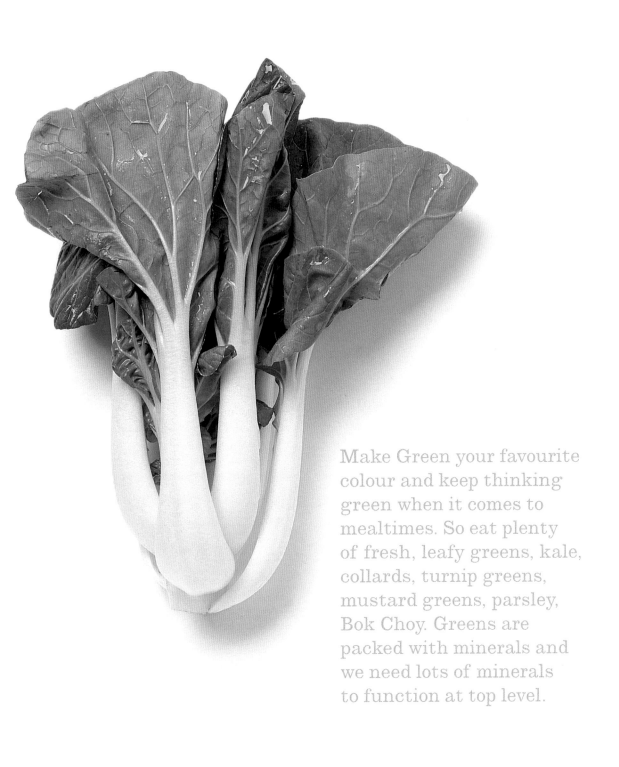

Make Green your favourite
colour and keep thinking
green when it comes to
mealtimes. So eat plenty
of fresh, leafy greens, kale,
collards, turnip greens,
mustard greens, parsley,
Bok Choy. Greens are
packed with minerals and
we need lots of minerals
to function at top level.

level three
the Dr Gillian detox

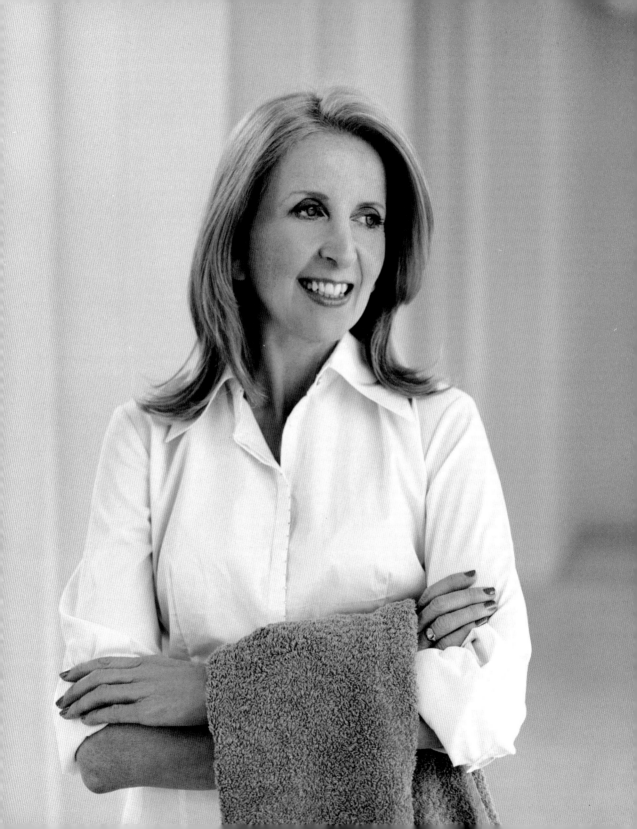

We hear about detox a lot. My message to you is that opting for a healthy lifestyle is more important than crash detoxing. Once you've followed my plan and are well in the groove, then a cleansing detox can be great once every few months. In this chapter I'll give you a really simple two-day detox you can try when you feel you want to.

Don't use detoxing as a substitute for a healthy diet.

A dear friend of mine from New York is the ultimate detox junkie. Barbara is often overweight and loves to gorge on hard cheeses – breakfast, lunch and dinner – sometimes eating very large slabs at one sitting. She tells me that when no-one is around she tucks into cakes, ice cream and anything that sounds, looks or smells like a crisp. She loves living in New York City because she says it is the one place where she can call in for a takeaway at any time of the day or night, or even pop out in the early hours to get a large of tub of cookies-and-cream ice cream which she has been known to wolf down at four in the morning.

When I confront Barbara about her eating habits, she tells me not to worry. She says that she actually is very health conscious because she detoxes on a regular basis at a centre in California. During these intervals, she eats nothing but bean sprouts and drinks gallons of cucumber juice. But I have since learned that she is not as goody-two-shoes as she would like us all to think. The last time I tried to contact her when she was at the centre in California, she had disappeared. No-one knew where she was. It turned out she had escaped in search of cherry pie and the next day had to order a colonic in the vain hope that she would redress the balance.

Barbara mistakenly believes that she can abuse her body at home, day in and day out, and then counteract the impact every few months with a severe detox. But it just doesn't work that way. Detoxes are fine, but not at the expense of a daily, healthy eating plan. But as part of a healthy lifestyle they are a fantastic way to cleanse and replenish.

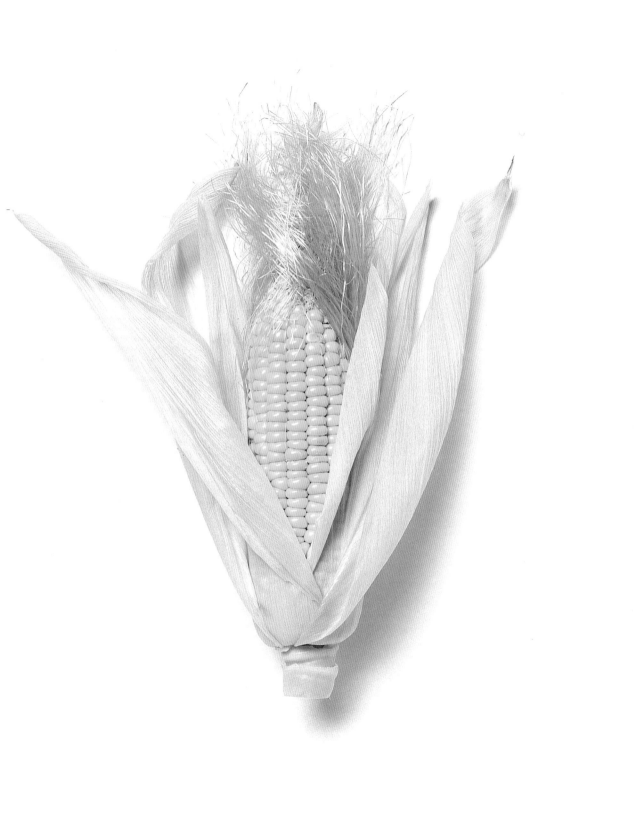

As part of a healthy lifestyle,
detoxes are a fantastic way
to cleanse and replenish.

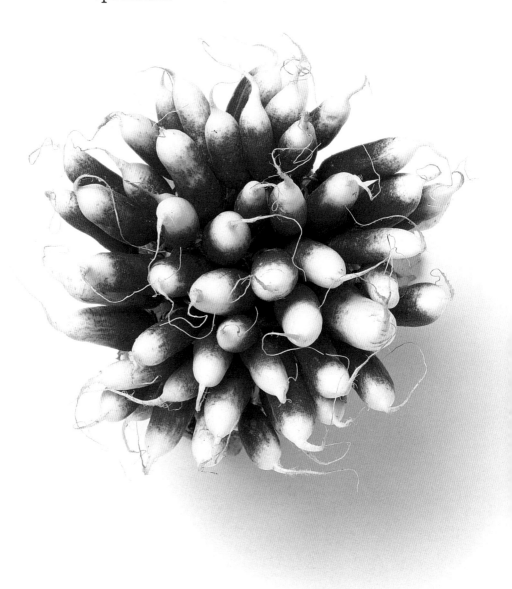

WHY DETOX AT ALL?

The body is naturally detoxing every day. However, depending on what you eat, how you live your life, where you live, and how your body performs, natural detoxing often needs some help.

The colon is the body's sewage system. If the sewage system stops flowing efficiently, toxins collect in the colon and become a breeding ground for unhealthy bacteria. Blood capillaries lining the colon wall begin to absorb toxins into the bloodstream and this lowers the overall performance of bodily functions. Over time, these toxins can build up in the body, settling in the various organs and causing fatigue, digestive problems, weight gain, and a variety of skin, hair and health problems.

TOP DETOX FOODS

Artichokes	Garlic	Radishes
Asparagus	Grapefruit	Raw cabbage
Broccoli	Green leaves	Raw food
Cauliflower	Hemp seeds (raw shelled)	Sprouted seeds
Chicory	Lemons	Tarragon
Daikon	Linseeds	Turmeric
Dandelion tea	Lovage	Veggie juices
Fennel	Mung beans	Warm water
Fruit salad	Nettle tea	Watermelon
Fruit smoothies	Papaya	

GETTING STARTED

Weekends are usually easier for a two-day detox. However, it is not set in stone that it must be over a weekend. Just make sure that it is carried out over two consecutive days.

YOUR DETOX KIT

1 Foods and teas for the cleanse
2 Juicer or a shop nearby that can make juices for you
3 Blender
4 Skin brush
5 Two candles
6 Essential oils of Myrrh and Frankincense
7 A notepad
8 Lots of still bottled water if you do not have a filter
(drink about 2 litres of water each day of the detox)
9 Linseeds
10 Hemp oil or Extra Virgin olive oil
11 Hot water bottle
12 Fun music to dance to and let go
13 Fresh mint
14 A cup of castor oil
15 Cotton sheeting
16 Powdered acidophilus

Early to Bed, Early to Rise

I want you in your bed early for a week before your detox and during the detox. No later than 10.30pm. Sleep is an essential part of the process.

Deep Breathing

On waking up, the day before your detox and during the two-day detox, sit on a hard-surfaced chair with your bare feet firmly planted on the floor.

► Feel the soles of the feet touching the surface of the floor
► Feel with the palm of your hand the area under your tummy button
► Place the palm of your hand flat on that area
► Close your eyes and relax
► Breathe deeply, then as you breathe out say: '*I am healthy. I eat good food every day.*'
► Repeat this affirmation 10 times

Bath Time

Take only short baths during the detox weekend. If you feel like having a hot bath make sure that it is a 20-minute bath at most.

The night before your detox, soak two tablespoons of organic linseeds in a large bowl of hot water.

Stay at home or close to home on your detox days.

Day 1

ON WAKING

Deep breathing exercise
(See page 165)

One cup of warm lemon and lime water
A cup of warm water is a cleansing way
to start the day. Add a few squeezes of lemon
and a couple of squeezes of lime for even
greater effect. Take your time to drink it.
There is no need to rush.

One small cup of Dandelion tea

Strain the linseeds that you have soaked
overnight and drink only the broth.

Exercise
Twenty-minute brisk walk.

Dry skin brush
Dry skin brushing speeds up the rate
at which toxins are expelled from the
body, because it stimulates blood cells
and lymph tissue, two key physiological
detoxification avenues.

Brush smoothly the soles of the feet,
working your way up the legs, then up
the arms and down the back. Brush in long
sweeping movements towards your heart,
as it increases circulation and improves skin
tone and texture. Always brush lightly and
gently, and avoid areas of broken skin,
thread veins and varicose veins.

Take your shower after skin brushing.

BREAKFAST

Large Fruit Salad Berry Compote
¹/₂ a small tub of blueberries
¹/₂ a small tub raspberries
¹/₂ a small punnet strawberries
Or more if you want

Berries are superb for the liver. Nourishing
the liver is key for detoxification.

1 mug of Dandelion tea

MID-MORNING
Turn on your favourite piece of music, dance and have fun.

Fruit Juice
**¹/₂ pineapple or more (simply pass
through the juicer and serve).**

Exercise
Before lunch, go for a brisk walk.

LUNCH

Warm Detox Broth

You are going to simmer these vegetables and drink only the broth. Please try to get organic vegetables whenever possible. Do not peel the veggies if they are organic.

6 carrots
3 large white potatoes
1 Daikon or 4 radishes
2 turnips
1 cup parsley
4 celery stalks
1 garlic clove
1 strip of kombu (seaweed)

1. Fill a saucepan with 2.5 litres of water. Pop your veggies into the pot and bring to the boil.
2. Reduce the heat, put a lid on the pot and simmer for 2 hours on a very low heat.
3. Strain the vegetables and drink a third of the broth. Save the rest for the evening and for tomorrow.

Detox Sprout Salad
SERVES 1
100g organic mung bean sprouts
40g celery, finely sliced
40g Chinese cabbage, shredded
Squeeze of lemon juice
6 chicory leaves

1. Place the sprouts, celery and cabbage in a salad bowl and mix well. Squeeze over the lemon juice.
2. Arrange the chicory leaves on a plate, spoon over the mung bean sprout salad and serve.

MID-AFTERNOON
Turn on your favourite piece of music and dance like crazy.

Vegetable Juice
6 carrots
1 cucumber
2 celery stalks
1/2 onion
handful of cabbage leaves

1 cup nettle tea

LATE AFTERNOON

Vegetable Juice
1 fennel
1 whole cucumber
2 celery sticks
(add a small piece of ginger if you feel cold and want warming up)

1 cup of nettle tea

Exercise
Before dinner, go for a brisk walk.

DINNER
Eat early, around 6pm.

Detox Broth (see page 167)
Raw Pâté with Sprouts

Fresh mint tea
Take a generous handful of fresh mint leaves
and steep in boiling water for a few minutes
before drinking

Raw Pâté
SERVES 2
2 tbsps torn fresh basil
1 tbsp chopped coriander
200g whole almonds, soaked
75g pine nuts
2 tbsps lemon juice
1 garlic clove

1. Place all ingredients in a food processor
and blend until smooth.
2. Place in a small bowl and refrigerate.
3. Serve with mixed sprouts.

Dry skin brush and a short bath

Apply castor oil pack
Using a castor oil pack seems to increase
detoxification through the liver and trigger
the organs of elimination to open and release.
It may also stimulate the lymphatics and
improve circulation and the removal of
toxins generally.

Find a piece of cotton fabric that,
when folded so that it is four layers thick,
will cover your abdomen from your hips to
your chest. You can tear up an old cotton
sheet for this. Fold the fabric into four and
pour castor oil liberally on to the top layer of
the fabric – about a cup of oil. Lie down and
place the castor oil pack over your abdomen
with the oiled layer of fabric against the
skin. Cover it with a towel or some plastic
wrap, for instance cling film, to prevent
the oil reaching any linen or clothing.

Apply a hot water bottle to the liver and
abdominal area. Hold in place for a minimum
of an hour. If the hot water bottle cools refill
with hot water. You need to keep it as hot
as possible for maximum benefits.

NOTE: PACKING WOULD NOT BE ADVISED DURING
MENSTRUATION, PREGNANCY OR LACTATION.

Meditation by candlelight

Place a white candle in a safe place so that it is about a foot in front of you. Make sure you can look at it without slouching or feeling uncomfortable. Sitting at a table is often the best position for this meditation.

Light the candle. Close your eyes and focus on your body and your centre. Ground yourself in the moment by being aware of the ground, floor, chair or whatever you are sitting on.

Open your eyes and look at the flame and pay attention to it – the colours, the movement, and the still place in the centre of it.

You'll have thoughts. Let them go without worrying about them and bring your attention back to the candle. Do this for about ten minutes.

The candle symbolically serves to represent the burning away of any negative energies you may have attracted and/or created.

DAY TWO PREP

Soak 2 tablespoons of organic linseeds in a large bowl of hot water.

For inspiration and motivation during the two-day detox, always remind yourself why you are embarking upon this cleansing programme. It's a chance for you to purge out toxic residues, take care of your body, glands, organs, cells and general health.

BEFORE BED

Drink a cup of warm water an hour before bed. Just before bed, get out your notepad and take time to write down your thoughts about today. How do you feel? What emotions do you have? Don't hold back. Write down everything that comes into your head.

Keep your notepad and pen by your bed. If you have any dreams tonight, write them down on waking.

10pm BEDTIME

Day 2

You are going to drink loads of juice during Day 2. I don't want you just to drink one or two juices, I want you to drink lots of juices to satisfy and cleanse your bowels, organs and cells. This is not about depriving yourself. If you feel, 'I want food, I'm hungry,' then please drink more juice. You should be able to satisfy your hunger cravings, if you have any, by simply drinking enough juice.

A full day of drinking just fresh juice is one of the most efficient ways to dislodge mucus and catarrh, cleanse the organs – especially the kidneys, liver and bowels – while simultaneously infusing nutrients and live enzymes into your body with the least amount of effort from your digestive system.

Obviously, if hunger and a dissatisfied feeling become overwhelming, then by all means please eat some solid vegetables or brown rice. It is not a problem if that's what you need to do the first time round.

You can consume one fruit smoothie and one fruit juice in the morning up until about 11am. After then swap to veggie juices. You might also buy some powdered acidophilus from a health store and drink towards the end of the day. The acidophilus will help to spur the growth of healthy bacteria. Drink the acidophilus with water.

A Word About the Juices

I want you to feel free to choose those vegetable juices that are right for you. If you find the taste of vegetable juices 'hard going', then simply add some carrot juice (or apple) to the vegetable juice. Because carrots are a sweet-tasting vegetable, they will soften the taste of any other more sour vegetable. Celery and cucumber juices tend to have more neutral flavours too.

I have included times in the second day. If possible do try to stick to these – as you'll see you've got a lot of juicing to get through!

7am ON WAKING

Deep Breathing Exercise (see page 165)

One cup of warm water with a squeeze of lemon and lime
1/2 cup nettle tea mixed with 1/2 cup slippery elm tea

Exercise
Go for a 20-minute brisk walk.

8am BREAKFAST

Strain the linseeds you have been soaking overnight from the water and drink only the liquid.

Fruit smoothie
4 peaches
2 pears
6 apricots
OR a nice big slice of watermelon if in season.

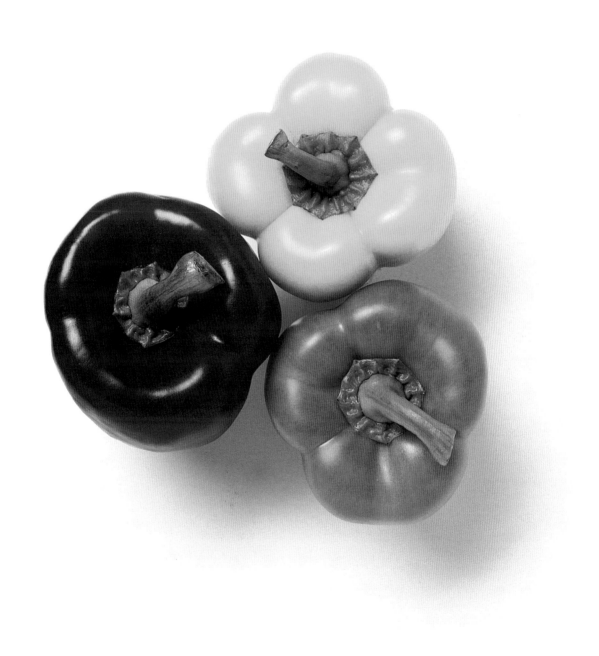

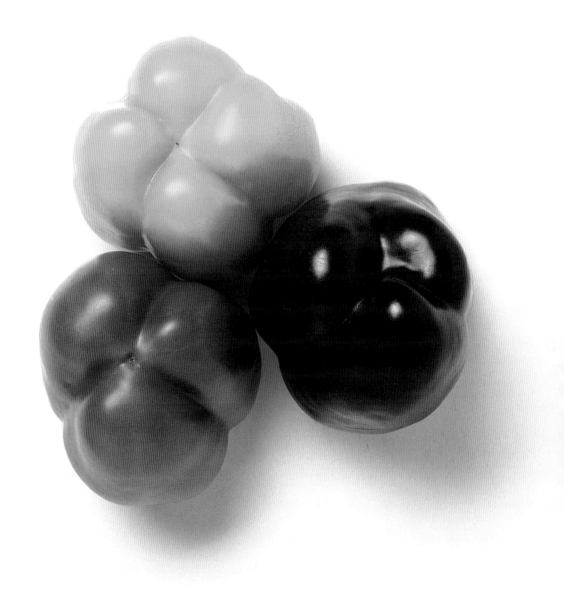

10:15am Vegetable juice
handful alfalfa sprouts
4 celery stalks
1 cucumber
3 broccoli florets
1 garlic bulb

11:15am Dandelion tea

11:30am Go for a 20-minute brisk walk

NOON

Juicy Detox Smoothie
6 carrots
1 celery
1 ripe avocado
1 apple
squeeze of lemon
8 basil leaves

1. Juice the apple, celery and carrots
through your juicer.
2. Place the juice in your blender
with the avocado and basil leaves.
3. Squeeze a dash of lemon into the
blend and serve.

2:15pm Vitality Juice
6 tomatoes
6 carrots
6 celery stalks
1 red pepper
½ beetroot
1 cucumber
¼ onion
¼ green cabbage head
6 green beans

4pm Vegetable juice (see Day One)

5pm Go for a 20- minute brisk walk

6pm Detox Broth (see Day One)

Detox Sprout Salad
SERVES 1
125g cucumber, finely sliced
50g beansprouts
30g watercress leaves (or baby spinach)
juice of half a lemon
2 tbsp fresh mint, chopped

1. Place the cucumber, sprouts, watercress
leaves and lemon juice in a bowl.
2. Pour over the lemon juice, sprinkle with
fresh mint and serve immediately.

8:30pm Detox Bath
Use a few drops of the myrrh and
frankincense oils in the bath. Remember
not to make your bath too hot or too long.
A 20-minute soak is just fine. Light some
candles in the bathroom and relax.

Early to bed, early to rise makes you healthy,
stealthy and wise!! Make sure that you get
early to bed for maximum rest. Fill your hot
water bottle with hot water. Lie down on your
bed with the hot water bottle placed above
your buttocks, in the lower and middle lower
area of your back. You are essentially
warming the kidneys and should feel pretty
relaxed too. Also, remember to drink a cup
of warm water an hour or so before bed.

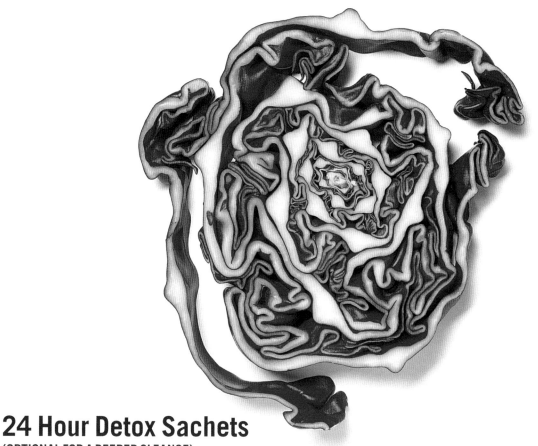

24 Hour Detox Sachets
(OPTIONAL FOR A DEEPER CLEANSE)

After years of working with people suffering from toxicity
and weight issues, I developed a combination powder formula
for liver, gall bladder and colon detox, available in health
foods shops. It works like a charm and my clients swear by it.
It will give you one of the best clean outs you have ever had.
But you will need to stay at home for 24 hours. My clients
call my 24 hour detox, 'A colonic without a tube up the
bahookee!' It consists of pumpkin seeds, papayas, lemon
balm, magnesium and oats.

DO YOU NEED ADRENAL CLEANSING?

Do you suffer from the following?

- ► Overweight
- ► Beer belly
- ► Middle Age spread
- ► Energy slumps mid-afternoon
- ► Difficulty getting out of bed
- ► Feeling constantly stressed

Poor adrenal function can hold back weight loss. It's important to give this gland a cleansing. My top tip is to take 15 drops of liquid Astragalus twice daily and a Vitamin B Complex, 50mg once a day for two months after the Detox. And for one month after that, take 15 drops of liquid Siberian Ginseng daily.

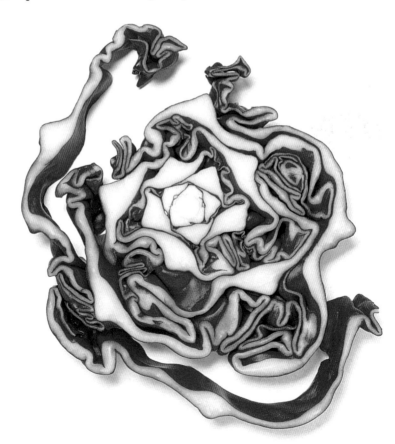

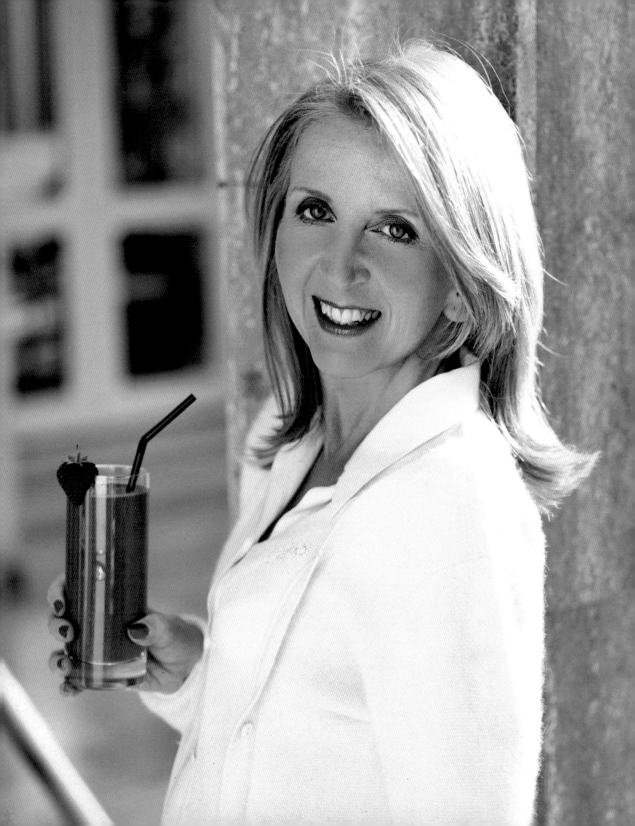

level four
slim for life

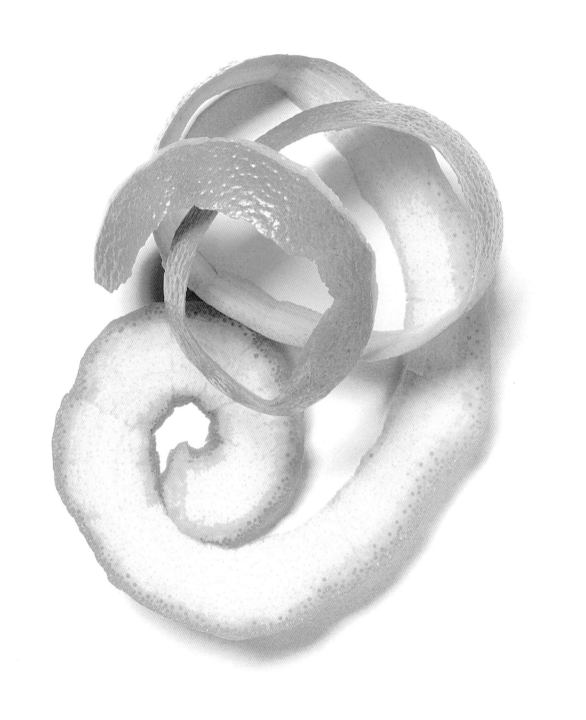

ASSESSMENT REPORT

At the very beginning of the book, I asked you to catalogue a seven-day food and drink inventory. You collected all your food packaging for a week and analysed the ingredients. You established your goals, banished your excuses, dumped your junk and flicked the healthy eating switch. This was my way of setting you on the right path and giving you a starting point for your journey.

In life, it is important to take special moments out to reflect on where you are. In other words, every so often it is helpful to look at the progress you are making. This process of reflection helps to motivate, inspire, encourage, foster hope, and also constructs a leaping-board from which to spring to your next level. Now is that time. I want you to review and assess the progress that you have made since your starting point.

Following the guidelines within my plan, develop your own seven-day programme. And while you follow your own plan, I want you to keep a diary of everything you eat and drink. After a week, compare your new diary with your original. I know you are going to see some amazing differences.

After that, I want you to complete the Self Assessment Form.

Self Assessment

1 What is the percentage of fresh food and vegetables in your diet now as opposed to before?

2 Are you now eating a greater variety of food groups and foods such as beans, whole grains, pulses, legumes, seeds, seaweeds?

3 How much raw food are you eating now versus before?

4 Are you drinking more water?

5 How much healthier are your snacks compared with at the beginning?

6 Have you substantially reduced your intake of red meat, wheat and milk products?

7 Have you drastically reduced or cut out the nasties – sugar, sweets, chocolate, caffeine, alcohol, table salt?

8 How do you feel? Are you healthier?

9 Look in the mirror. What has changed about your body?

10 Do you have more energy now?

11 Is your digestion better?

12 Are you sleeping well?

13 Do you have more confidence preparing your own foods?

14 Are you exercising regularly?

15 Are you feeling happier, slimmer and sexier?

HOW WOULD YOU RATE YOUR OVERALL GENERAL PROGRESS?

These are questions for you to ponder. I am not looking for you to score anything. I just want you to reflect within your own self by yourself.

EXCELLENT PROGRESS You are doing Fab!
GOOD PROGRESS Hang in there.
SATISFACTORY PROGRESS Could do better.
NO PROGRESS Back to the drawing board.
You need my SOS Emergency Plan (page 206).

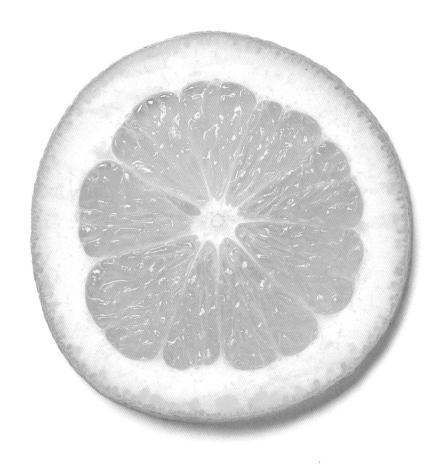

THE 90/10 RULE

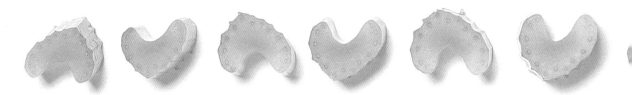

I have been called a stick in the mud, a party pooper, a food fascist and the Diet Dictator! Yes, I am tough and that's not going to change. I want you to get fantastic results. The bottom line is that I want you to get well and be healthier than you have ever known. I want you to reach your desired weight. And I know what it takes to get you there. It requires determination, willpower, drive and a willingness to change.

During the plan I've owned you, but once you graduate you can move on to bigger and better things. After the eight weeks, I won't bop you over the head if you are compelled to deviate a tiny bit. Once you have proven yourself during my eight-week boot camp, I no longer require a full 100 per cent compliance. I call it my 90/10 Rule.

I used to tell my clients to use my 80/20 rule but I am now modifying that advice. Much to my chagrin, I have learned that some people are carefully working out how 20 per cent of their meals can be bad. So I have decided to shift the percentages slightly, to 90/10. This way, there is less room for negative manoeuvering.

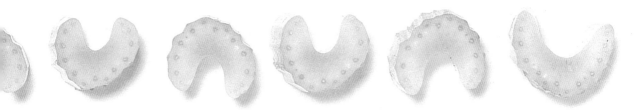

It's Not About a Calculation

I am only talking figuratively. The 90/10 rule is nothing to do with numbers or calculations. Ultimately I want you to live the lifestyle 100 per cent of the time but I do also realize that at certain times, it may not be possible or desirable.

For example, you may go out for a date on a Saturday night and the restaurant has great desserts on offer and you want one of them. Go ahead and order it. Or you may have ordered a soup made with cream. It's OK to eat it. You may be on a long drive in the car where you have to stop at a motorway rest stop and they only have roasted nuts instead of raw. I don't want you to say, 'Oh I can't have that.' The fact is, if you are hungry by all means go for the best of what you can get at that moment. It's okay because we have established that there is a figurative 90/10 rule. Do not feel guilty or beat yourself up over it because you now know that there is a guilt-free window of opportunity, albeit a small one.

What I don't want you to do is to calculate that 10 per cent of your meals should be bad food. This would be the opposite of my intention. I would be horrified to think that you are trying to calculate bad food into your regimen. My intention is that you live the lifestyle and do the best that you are able. So it's important to focus on the 90 per cent.

Treats can be Goodies

Most people think that treats have to be bad for you. They have a point; most conventional treats are loaded with sugar, fat and chemicals. Since childhood we get conditioned to think these treats taste good.

People are always terrified that there won't be any treats on my Plan. Not so. First, check out my *You Are What You Eat Cookbook* (Michael Joseph) which has full chapters on healthy and delicious treats, snacks and quick bites.

I want you to change the mental association you might have with treats. As a child, you may have received sweets from parents, grandparents, aunts. Your brain makes an association with the taste of the treat and a feeling of love, giving and happiness. It can leave an imprint for a lifetime, meaning that you then go after these treats to make you feel warm and loved again.

And to add insult to injury, sweets such as chocolate actually contain some ingredients that release feel-good chemicals in the brain. As a result, it is easy to fall into that treat trap.

If you think you might associate treats like cake and chocolate with feelings of happiness or comfort, then now is the perfect time to acknowledge it. You now know that foods laden with bad fats and refined sugars are far from good for you, so it's time to enjoy a whole new set of treats.

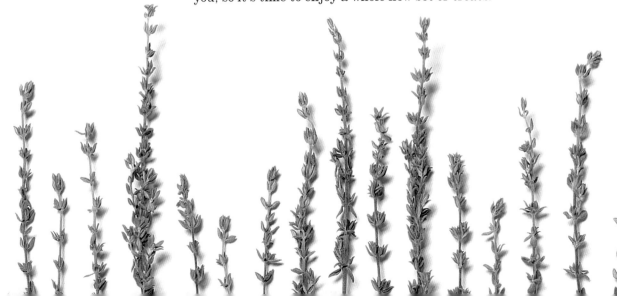

Treats that Won't Send you Back to Level One

Let me tell you a little story about treats. The other day
I was on the train to the airport. I sat next to a woman who was
delightedly tucking into a great big chocolate croissant with
a mountain of whipped cream on top. Totally oblivious to my
presence just inches away, she was savouring every crumb, but
just as she was about to indulge in her last bite, she casually
glanced around and caught my eye. She looked away, looked
nervously down at her crumbs, and then did a double take.

PASSENGER: Oh My God, it's you! I can't believe
you're sitting next to me in the train. I watch your show.
GILLIAN: So why did you eat that rubbish?
PASSENGER: I don't do this all the time.
GILLIAN: Was that your breakfast?
PASSENGER: Yes. But it was just a little treat.

I don't do, 'Yes buts.' I do, however, have lots of alternatives
to offer you. Treats do not need to be filled with sugar, chocolate,
wheat, additives, chemicals and synthetic creams. When you
eat these kinds of foods, generally you are going to feel horrible
either right afterwards, shortly afterwards, or in the long-term.
It's a guarantee that you will affect your body negatively and
most likely feel it. Eat my healthy treats and you will feel good.
No guilt trip necessary.

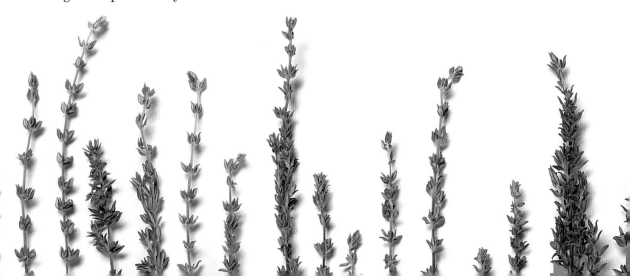

GILLIAN'S ULTIMATE HEALTH TREATS

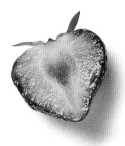 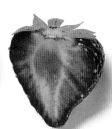 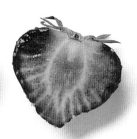 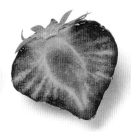 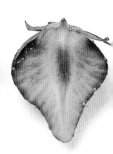

Sweet

- ▶ Fresh fruit such as: grapes, strawberries, blueberries, peaches
- ▶ Fruit salad
- ▶ Fruit smoothies
- ▶ Dried figs
- ▶ Prunes
- ▶ Medjool dates
- ▶ Natural organic yoghurt, but it must be free of added sugar and sweeteners

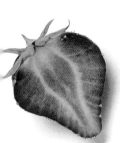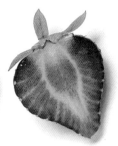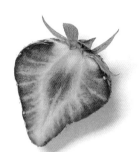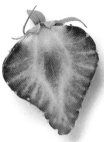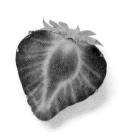

Baked Apples (or Pears)

1. Preheat oven to 200C/Gas 6.
2. Place 2 apples in an ovenproof dish.
3. Bake for 15–20 minutes.

Baked Figs with Agave and Lemon

SERVES 1
2 figs cut in half
1/2 tbsp agave syrup
juice of 1/2 lemon
1 star anise (optional)

1. Preheat the oven to 180C/Gas 4.
2. Take a large piece of foil and place the halved figs in the centre, pour over the syrup and lemon juice and add the star anise if using.
3. Scrunch up the foil and place on a baking sheet.
Place in the oven and bake for 20 minutes.
4. Remove from the oven and allow to stand for 5 minutes.
Serve from the foil.

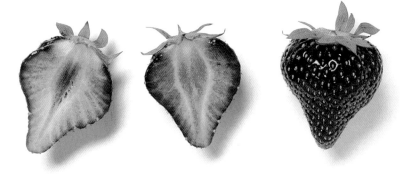

Strawberry Ice

For best results use an ice-cream maker. Alternatively freeze in a shallow plastic container and whisk every 30 minutes with a fork until the mixture has frozen. It works well with raspberries too. Great treat for the kids.

MAKES 1 LITRE
500g fresh hulled strawberries plus extra to garnish
2 tbsp agave syrup
500ml rice milk
mint leaves to garnish

1. Place the strawberries in the food processor or blender and blend until smooth. Add the agave syrup and rice milk and blend for a further 30 seconds.
2. Pour into an ice cream-maker and leave to churn for 20 to 30 minutes.
3. Scoop into a glass dish and garnish with fresh fruit and mint leaves.

Mango Granita

This healthy reward will keep well in the freezer for up to
a month, so it is worth making up a batch when mangos are
ripe and inexpensive. Allow to thaw for 5 to 10 minutes at
room temperature before serving

2 ripe mangos
juice of 1 lime
100 ml cold water
4 bunches fresh redcurrants

1. With a sharp knife cut the cheeks from the sides of the
mangos. Cut these in half and then slide the knife blade under
the skin to remove the flesh. Trim as much flesh from the stone
as possible and place all of it in the food processor or blender.
2. Blend until you have a smooth pulp. Add the lime juice and
water and process for a further 15 seconds.
3. Turn the puree into a plastic container and place
in the freezer.
4. Every 30 minutes whisk the mixture vigorously with a fork.
The sorbet should be ready in 2–3 hours and should appear
quite grainy in texture.
5. Serve in tall-stemmed glasses garnished with fresh
redcurrants or other fruit.

Rhubarb Crumble

When cooking fruits such as rhubarb, do not allow the fruit to boil. It should simply cook at a low simmer. This will ensure as many of the nutrients as possible are preserved. Rhubarb is an excellent source of calcium.

SERVES 2
100g rhubarb, chopped
½ tbsp agave syrup
75ml cold water
FOR THE TOPPING
50g porridge oats
½ tbsp millet flour
1 tbsp agave syrup

1. Place the rhubarb, agave syrup and water in a small pan. Cook over a gentle heat for 15 minutes. Remove from the heat, allow to cool slightly and then transfer to a small pie dish.
2. Preheat the oven to 180C/Gas 4.
3. Place the oats and flour in a mixing bowl and stir well. Then mix in the syrup. The mixture will appear a little lumpy.
4. Scatter the mixture over the fruit. Do not press the mixture down.
5. Transfer to the oven and bake for 15 minutes until the top is crisp.
6. Remove from the oven and allow to stand for 5 minutes before serving.

Date and Almond Truffles

8 fresh dates
100g ground almonds
2 tsp carob powder
finely grated rind and freshly squeezed juice of lime
Macadamia nuts or Brazil nuts (optional)
chopped mixed nuts (optional)

1. Place the dates, almonds, carob powder,
lime rind and juice into a food processor.
2. Blend until the mixture forms a stiff ball.
3. Add more lime juice if necessary to help bring
the mixture together.
4. Remove blade and roll date mixture into balls.
Place in truffle cases or roll in chopped, mixed nuts.
5. Fill each with a Macadamia or Brazil nut.
6. Cover and keep in the fridge.

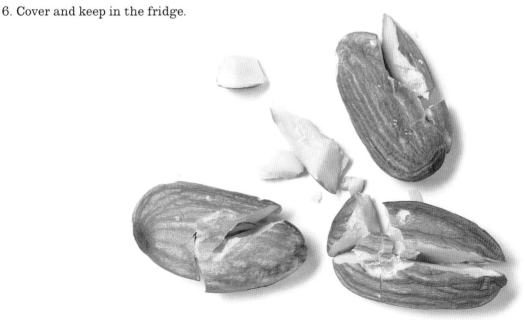

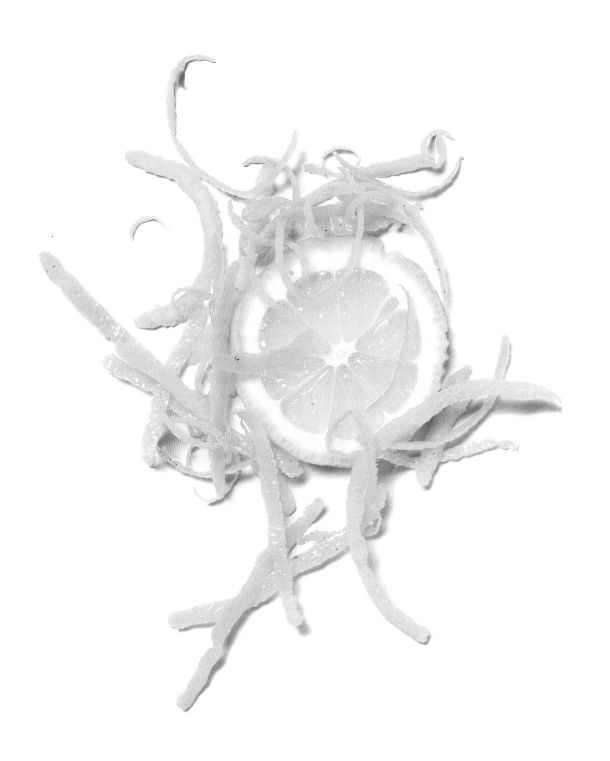

Lemon Tofu Chiffon Cake

349g pack firm silken tofu
3 tbsp agave syrup
Rind of 2 lemons plus juice of 2
100g gram or chickpea flour
2 tsp baking powder
2 tbsp water

1. Preheat the oven to 170C/Gas 3. Line a 500g loaf tin
with baking parchment.
2. Place the tofu, syrup, lemon rind and juice in a mixing
bowl and beat with an electric mixer until smooth and light.
This will take 5 minutes.
3. Mix the baking powder and flour together and beat into
the tofu 2 tbsp at a time. Whisk with the mixer for a further
5 minutes.
4. Transfer to the prepared tin and bake for 25–30 minutes
until firm but still springy to the touch. Remove from the oven
and allow to cool slightly and then lift out with the baking
parchment and allow to cool completely.
5. Serve in slices.

Carrot Cake

Agave syrup happens to taste sweet and comes from
the cactus plant.

100g grated carrot
2 oranges
4 tbsp agave syrup
1 free range egg
150g gram or chickpea flour
1/2 tsp baking powder
100g soft silken tofu

1. Preheat the oven to 170C/Gas 3. Line a 500g loaf tin
with baking parchment.
2. Grate the orange zest. Place the carrot, zest of 1 1/2 oranges
half the syrup in a mixing bowl. Stir with a fork and make
a well in the centre.
3. Break the egg into the well and whisk the egg until light
and frothy.
4. Mix the flour with the baking powder and then beat into
the carrot mixture 2 tablespoonfuls at a time.
5. Add the juice of 1 orange and mix well. Place half the juice
of the second orange in the base of the loaf tin.
6. Transfer the carrot mixture to the prepared tin and smooth
the surface with a pallet knife. Place in the preheated oven and
bake for 25–30 minutes or until well risen, golden in colour and
firm to the touch.
7. Remove from the oven and lift the cake out of the tin using
the parchment. Allow to cool.
8. Beat the tofu with the remaining syrup until light and
smooth, then add the juice of 1/2 an orange. Stir well to mix
and leave to stand for a few minutes.
9. When the cake is cold top with the frosting, sprinkle over
the remaining zest and serve.

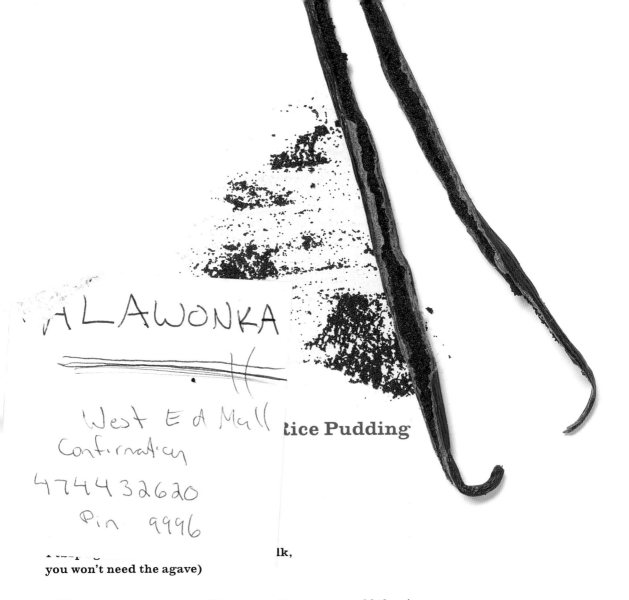

ALAWONKA

West Ed Mall
Confirmation
474432620
Pin 9996

Rice Pudding

lk,
you won't need the agave)

1. Place the water or rice milk in a small saucepan, add the rice, cinnamon, vanilla, orange zest and juice and the syrup if using.
2. Bring to the boil, cover and simmer for 25–30 minutes, stirring occasionally.

Carob Mousse

SERVES 4

4 tsp carob powder
4 tsp very hot water
240g soft silken tofu
4 tsp rice syrup
4 tsp agave syrup
6 drops pure vanilla essence
freshly ground cinnamon to taste
4 sprigs of mint to garnish

1. Place the carob in a small bowl, add the hot water
and mix well until the carob powder has dissolved.
2. Place the tofu in a medium-sized bowl and whisk
with a balloon whisk or electric whisk until it is smooth.
3. Beat the liquid carob mixture into the tofu, then beat
in the rice syrup followed by the agave syrup. Whisk
well between each addition.
4. Add the vanilla essence and cinnamon, whisk just
to combine then transfer to 4 small glasses or glass dishes.
5. Chill for 30 minutes or up to 2 hours. Serve garnished
with a sprig of mint.

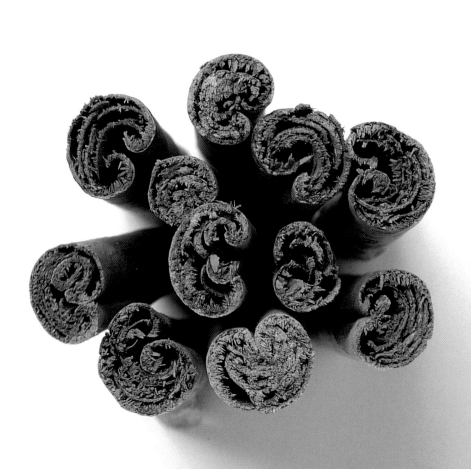

Savoury

- Vegetable juices
- Oatcakes
- Rice cakes with mashed avocado, houmous, dill and topped off with tomato halves
- Vegetable crudités with houmous or other healthy dips (see page 200)
- Soaked almonds or soaked nuts of any sort (soaking nuts overnight always makes them easier to digest and sweeter tasting)
- Nuts
- Steamed nuts
- Raw shelled hemp seeds mashed into avocados
- Raw shelled hemp seeds with anything!
- Roasted sweet potatoes with mashed avocados and herbs such as basil
- Shitake mushrooms on wheat-free toast
- Sautéed pumpkin seeds with wheat-free Tamari sauce

Baked Beetroot

Preheat oven to 200C/Gas 6
Wrap in foil and bake for 30 minutes

Baked Sweet Potatoes

Preheat oven to 200C/Gas 6
Wrap in foil and bake for 30 minutes

Baked and Sliced Butternut Squash

Preheat oven to 200C/Gas 6
Wrap in foil and bake for 45 minutes

Baked Yams

Preheat oven to 200C/Gas 6
Wrap in foil and bake for 30 minutes

Calzone with Cherry Tomatoes and Courgettes

If it's pizza that you miss, then try these. You need to take a little care with the pastry or it will break up. If it does, don't worry too much, just press it back together.

MAKES 4
275g cherry tomatoes halved
1 bunch spring onions finely chopped
1 tbsp water (for tomato sauce)
2 tbsp freshly chopped basil
1 tbsp fresh oregano
200g buckwheat flour
2 tsp baking powder
2 tsp olive oil
150ml water (for pastry)
100g courgette cut into 1cm slices
fresh rocket to garnish

1. Place the cherry tomatoes, spring onions and water in a small pan and simmer gently over a low heat for 5–6 minutes. Remove from the heat and allow to cool then mix in the herbs.
2. Preheat the oven to 200C/Gas 6.
3. Mix the flour and baking powder in a bowl. Make a well in the centre, add the oil and 100ml of the water. Mix gently adding more water as required to make a soft dough.
4. Knead gently on a floured clean surface and divide the dough into 4 pieces and roll them out to form circles.
5. Divide the tomato mixture between the dough circles and top with the courgette slices. Carefully fold the dough over to form half moon shapes.
6. Transfer to a baking tin lined with parchment paper and bake for 10–12 minutes.
7. Remove from the oven and allow to cool for 5 minutes, before serving with the rocket garnish.

Dips

Spinach Dip

1 avocado, peeled and stone removed
juice of 1/2 lemon
225g can organic chickpeas, drained
200g fresh spinach

1. Place the avocado in the bowl of the processor with the lemon juice and chickpeas and process until you have a smooth paste.
2. Place the spinach in a steamer and steam for 1–2 minutes until just wilted. Remove from the heat and allow to cool slightly. Drain, then squeeze the spinach with your hand or the back of a spoon to remove any excess liquid.
3. Add the spinach to the avocado and chickpeas and process for a few seconds to combine. Transfer to a bowl and serve.

Cucumber and Garlic Dip

349g pack soft tofu
3–4 cloves garlic, peeled
handful of fresh mint leaves
1/4 cucumber, finely diced
lemon juice to taste

1. Place the tofu in the bowl of the food processor and process until smooth.
2. With the motor running add the garlic and then the mint leaves.
3. Transfer the mixture to a bowl and stir in the cucumber and some lemon juice to taste.
4. Serve immediately.

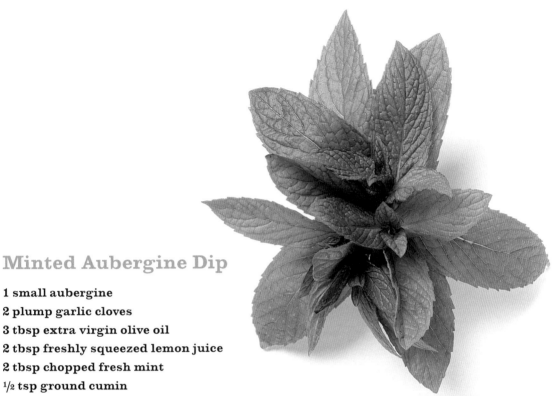

Minted Aubergine Dip

1 small aubergine
2 plump garlic cloves
3 tbsp extra virgin olive oil
2 tbsp freshly squeezed lemon juice
2 tbsp chopped fresh mint
¹/₂ tsp ground cumin

1. Preheat the oven to 200C/Gas 6.
2. Halve the aubergine. Peel the garlic and cut each clove into 4–5 slices.
3. Make a few deep incisions into the cut side of each aubergine half and place a slice of garlic well into each one.
4. Place aubergine halves on a baking tray and drizzle with 1 tbsp of the olive oil. Bake, cut side up, for 35–45 minutes until very tender and pale golden brown.
5. Remove from the oven and leave for about 20 minutes until cool enough to handle.
6. Using a dessertspoon, scoop the aubergine centre and softened garlic into a food processor, discarding the skin. Add the remaining olive oil, lemon juice, mint and cumin. Blend until smooth.

Non-Edible Treats

Treat yourself in different ways too. Try these ideas or create
your own luxury moments.

- **A sauna**
- **A swim**
- **A massage**
- **A facial**
- **A reflexology session**
- **Find a quiet space for meditation**
- **Watch a film**
- **Buy a new CD or DVD**
- **Treat yourself to a new outfit**
- **Read a good novel**
- **Take up a new hobby like tennis, squash, Tai Chi,
  kick boxing, dancing, Chi Kung, ice skating
  or whatever takes your fancy.**

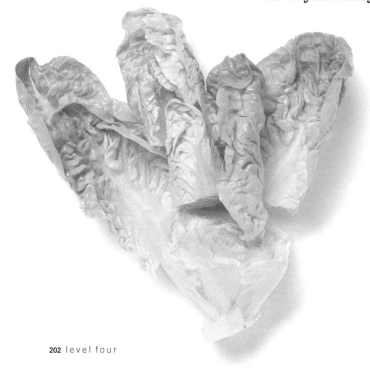

A Quick Guide to Eating Out

The first rule of eating out is to enjoy yourself. If you eat out regularly then you do need to be more careful, but if it's an occasional treat then I wouldn't want you to feel guilt over the salad dressing on the way home.

In restaurants, don't take it to extremes and don't try to force others to make the same choices as you. You want to be able to enjoy your time out and so do your dining partners. Here are a few guidelines to help keep eating out healthy, delicious and enjoyable:

▸ Don't starve yourself in anticipation of a restaurant meal. You are not on a calorie controlled diet.

▸ Twenty minutes before you eat, drink a glass of still water with no ice. You'll feel fuller and will digest the meal better. You can have little sips of water during the meal but no beer or fizzy drinks.

▸ Order first, so you won't be tempted or swayed by other people's (possibly unhealthy) choices. You may even set the stage for healthy eating for all.

▸ Order a vegetarian-based soup for starters, if possible. Try to avoid the dairy cream-based soups, and ask that cream not be added. Most soups will fill you up and are easy to digest. They are a great wholesome choice when eating out.

▸ Stop eating when you are two-thirds full. Listen to the cues your body gives you. It takes a while for your stomach's messages to get through to the brain, hence that 'over-stuffed' feeling you might get. You don't have to leave your plate empty. Ask how dishes are prepared. Waiters are becoming accustomed to these types of questions so don't worry about asking. Here are some of the questions you might want to pose:
Are your dishes baked? (good)
Are they grilled? (good)
Are they prepared with butter? (bad)
Or oil? (fine if not fried)
Is the fish wild? (good) Or farmed? (bad)
Ask what's in the sauce; ask what's in the soup; ask what's in the dressing. Excessive sugar and too much salt is what you are trying to avoid.

- Take your time. Put your knife and fork down between each bite. Take no notice of how quickly others may be eating.

- You can ask for the gravy, sauce or salad dressing to be served on the side. That way, if you don't like it or it comes laden with butter or sugar, it has not spoiled your meal. You can always ask for a lemon to squeeze over your fish or salad instead. But don't worry too much if the sauce or dressing is an integral part of the dish.

- Feel free to order two starters, or a starter and then a salad or combination of side dishes – not including fries! For example, I might have an artichoke heart salad to start and a combination of green beans, spinach and almond rice as my main course.

- If going out to a Chinese, Japanese or Thai restaurant make sure they do not use MSG (Monosodium glutamate) in their dishes.

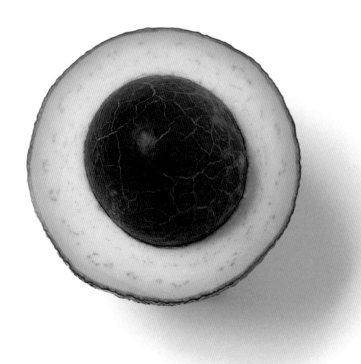

If you are ordering pasta, go for a tomato-based sauce rather than a cream-based sauce. Simpler dishes are often the most delicious.

Order off-menu if you have to. You could ask for grilled fish with vegetables and a salad made with oil and no butter. Or you could ask the chef what he/she can do for a vegetarian/vegan meal. Can he create something that is meat and dairy free? What can he come up with?

If you're thinking about dessert, wait about 10 minutes after finishing your main meal before ordering. Give your stomach time to tell your brain if it has had enough. If you still can't resist the chocolate delight, you can always split the dessert with your dining partner and let them eat the lion's share. Often a few bites are enough to satisfy.

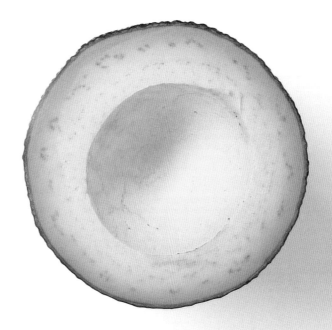

Dr Gillian's SOS Emergency Plan

If you've noticed yourself wandering off the path a few
too many times then you may need a jump-start. After all,
you don't want to go hurtling back to Level One.

DAY 1

If you have gone off the rails, don't fret. The last thing
I want you to feel is that it's game over, and you might as
well slip all the way down the slope and forget about healthy
eating altogether. It's easy to come back. Every day is a brand
new day where you can start again. And most important of
all, YOU ARE NOT ON A DIET. So you cannot fall off the diet,
fall off the wagon or eat too many calories. There's nothing
to fall off. When you picked up this book, it was to embark on
a lifestyle change. That is a completely different concept from
going on a diet. As one person put it on my website forum,
'Gillian's way is a state of mind. It is not a diet and therefore
not something that you can stop.'

I do demand that you embrace this healthy lifestyle as wholly
as you can and commit to it 100 per cent. But if something crazy
happens in your life and you veer off, so what? Don't worry about
it. Just keep doing what you set out to do. Keep embracing
the lifestyle. So if last Monday you missed breakfast and ate
a croissant in the middle of the day, you have not failed.

- ► **Acknowledge it**
- ► **Recognize it**
- ► **Take note of it**
- ► **Use it as a marker to stay on the path**

On Day One of your SOS Plan, the party you were invited to is off. The After-Work-Drinks-Meeting is postponed. I need your focus, effort and resolve.

Drink a cup of warm water with a squeeze of lemon right now. Then make sure that you drink another cup one hour before bed. Drink eight cups of warm water and plenty of herbal teas during the next three days. To get it all in, one rule of thumb is to drink one glass per hour. The only two teas I want you to drink today are Nettle or Dandelion. Take your pick. No moaning. I don't want to hear it.

Photocopy the SOS Emergency Exercise. You are going to use this for the next three days. Carry it with you wherever you go. Every two hours you will need to conduct the Emergency Exercise. It does not matter where you are, you could be on the plane, train, bus, at your desk in the office, in the kitchen, wherever.

Dr Gillian's SOS Emergency Exercise

1. Close your eyes.
2. Listen to your breath.
3. Count up from 1 to 10.
4. Repeat slowly the following words ten times, to yourself silently, or aloud. 'I live my new Lifestyle for life.'
5. At the end of the ten repetitions, visualise a movie screen with you in the lead role. In this film, you view a full day of your life acting out the lifestyle. So, for example, you see yourself eating a healthy breakfast; you witness yourself doing a 20-minute walk before a meal; you eat a fabulously healthy lunch and so on. At the end of the day in the movie, you see yourself happy, content and harmonised. And you are fully on track.
6. Count back down from 10 to 1.
7. Slowly open your eyes.

Day 1

MANTRA

Write the following statement 10 times: **I promise to eat breakfast**

BREAKFAST

Go out to your local supermarket and buy
a large fresh fruit salad already prepared
or make your own. That will be your
breakfast. Easy.

Chop up some raw fresh vegetables
or buy them already pre-chopped from
a supermarket. Get a selection of cucumbers,
carrots, red or yellow peppers, chicory,
mangetout. Take them to work and eat them
before, during and after lunch as snacks.
You can dip them in houmous.

LUNCH

Miso Soup. That's what you are having.
Buy it from a health food store. Pour the
packet into a mug and add hot water.
Have two mugs of miso soup.

AFTER WORK

Go home, turn on the radio to your
favourite station and dance like crazy.
Jump up and down, yell, sing out loud.
But most important, get moving.
(See page 74 for other exercise ideas.)

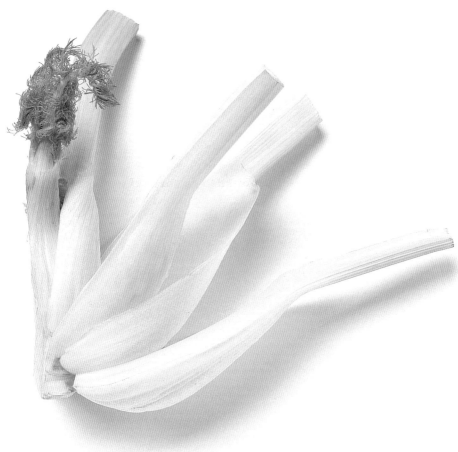

DINNER

After exercise, you must have a vegetable juice and follow it with a crunchy salad with sauerkraut and lemon squeezed over. If you live near a place that makes fresh vegetable juices, go and buy the juice. If not, make it yourself. It will take five minutes and is well worth the small effort.

SOS Juice

4 carrots
1/2 apple
2 celery sticks
1 cucumber
Tiny piece of ginger

Get to bed by 10pm for the next three days.

So you got through Day One. Well done. Now it's on to Day Two.

Plan your exact food menu in advance for the next day, I have given you space below to do this. To make it even easier for you, all you have to do is choose from the list provided on page 212. Advance planning is critical to staying on board. You will notice that much of the food is raw/uncooked, so preparation is minimal.

Day 2

DATE:

MANTRA
Write out the following statement 10 times: **I am on track with Gillian.**

BREAKFAST

SNACK

SNACK

DINNER

LUNCH

EXERCISE

Day 3

DATE:

MANTRA

Write out the following 10 times: **I am on track and I promise to eat breakfast.**

BREAKFAST

SNACK

SNACK

DINNER

LUNCH

EXERCISE

BREAKFAST CHOICES

Start each day with one cup of warm water with a squeeze of lemon juice, followed by a cup of nettle tea then choose from:

Apple/pear/peach/pineapple salad
2 pink grapefruit

Strawberry Banana Smoothie
Simply blend one punnet of strawberries, one ripe banana and 100ml water until smooth.

Millet Oat Porridge
It's comforting and creamy and tastes like oatmeal but with a fluffy, soothing texture.

50g millet flakes
50g oat flakes
400ml water

1. Bring the millet, oats and water to the boil in a pan.
2. Lower the heat and simmer for 3–5 minutes, stirring until you get the desired consistency. Sprinkle with dried herbs or a pinch of sea salt and serve.

It only takes minutes so no excuses now.

SNACKS FOR MID-MORNING

Choose from the following:
Apple
Pear
Grapes
Pineapple juice
Pink grapefruit juice
Vegetable juice. Either make your own and take it with you in a flask or buy one that is organic with no added sugar.

SNACKS FOR MID-AFTERNOON

Choose from the following:
At least a cup or more of crunchy sugar-snap peas
Handful of raw, unsalted Brazil nuts
Vitality Juice (page 173)

LUNCH CHOICES

Miso Soup with tofu
Chop a small slab of tofu into bite size cubes and throw into the soup.

Any kind of bean, vegetable or miso soup (either make your own or buy a sugar free veggie soup).
Follow the soup with a crunchy, green leafy salad.

DINNER

Appetiser: MUST HAVE vegetable juice
1 whole baby gem lettuce
6 celery stalks
1 fennel
1 cucumber
1 apple (optional for sweetness)

Baked Sweet Potato with Avocado and Warm Vegetable Salad

Get your taste buds ready for a hot baked sweet potato with a kick of cumin to satisfy any little cravings, buttery sliced avocado, fresh peppery leaves and warm vegetables – my ultimate feel-good foods.

SERVES 1
1 medium sweet potato – around 250g
½ yellow pepper
4 cherry tomatoes
1tsp olive oil
2 large handfuls wild rocket leaves
½ ripe avocado
Cress (optional)
Ground cumin to taste
DRESSING
1 tbsp olive oil
1 tsp organic balsamic vinegar
½ crushed clove garlic

1. Wash the potato and dry with kitchen paper. Place on a baking tray and cook in a preheated oven at 200C/Gas 6 for about 40 minutes until tender.
2. Thinly slice the yellow pepper and cut the cherry tomatoes in half.
3. Remove the tray from the oven and add the pepper and tomatoes. Drizzle with 1 tsp olive oil and return to the oven for five minutes.

4. Place the wild rocket leaves in a bowl and top with the sliced ripe avocado. Snip a little cress – if you have some handy – and sprinkle on top. Remove the potato and vegetables from the oven.
5. Place the potato on a plate, split it open and sprinkle with a good pinch of ground cumin. Scatter the warmed pepper and tomatoes over the salad. Toss together very lightly. Drizzle with 1 tbsp olive oil and 1 tsp organic balsamic vinegar mixed with half a crushed garlic clove. Serve with the hot potato.

EASY DINNER OPTIONS

1. Baked beans on wheat-free toast. Health food stores carry sugar free and sweetener free versions of baked beans. Serve with parsnip mash. Boil parsnips and mash with a little olive oil. If you can't get parsnips, use swedes, turnips, yams or squash. Add some baby gem lettuce and sprinkle with torn basil and chopped coriander.
2. Wheat-free pasta from a health food store or supermarket. Purchase an organic sugar-free sauce for pasta. Health food stores carry tomato-free sauces too. Toss with torn fresh basil leaves.
3. Tray of grilled veggies on a bed of green leaves. Slice and place a beet, a parsnip, onion, peppers, aubergine or courgette on a tray and drizzle with oil and a sprinkling of dried herbs. Simply grill and serve with fresh salad leaves and fresh basil.

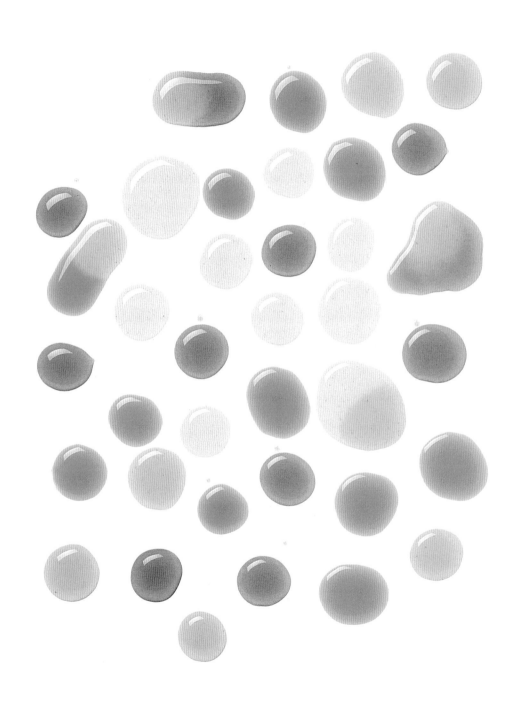

WHY MY SOS EMERGENCY PLAN WORKS

This mini plan I have devised is simple and uncomplicated.
It's enough for you to stay on track, while also addressing
your comfort needs. It's all of the following:

- **Easy**
- **Comforting**
- **Quick**
- **You will not feel hungry**
- **Inexpensive**
- **Uncomplicated**
- **A cinch**
- **Something to look forward to**
- **Enjoyable**
- **Focused**

You will feel better almost immediately on two levels: physically
and mentally. You are treating your body with the respect that
it deserves and you have taken definitive, positive steps. You will
now have the incentive to keep going over the long term, and you
should notice that you have more energy, are less bloated and
have the motivation to carry on with the lifestyle. You have not
fallen by the wayside. You are on track. The sky is the limit
with the results you can achieve.

Dr Gillian's Final Word for Ultimate Health

So now you know what to do. You have the tools for ultimate health. If you follow my plan, there are no failures. I truly hope that I have turned you on to the amazing possibilities that simple changes in eating and lifestyle can bring. I want you to feel fabulous now and for life. Here are some final words of advice I want to share with you . . .

Point One You need to care about what goes into your mouth. What you put in, is what you will get out. Put in good food, and you will feel the benefits. Food is energy, so fill up on the good stuff. Think about how well your body will run on pure, natural foods versus artificial foods empty of any real nutrition, taste or energy.

Point Two Food is one type of energy; your thoughts are also crucial points of energy. Keep your thoughts pure and positive. Like the food you eat, what you put into your head also affects your whole make-up. Fill yourself with happy thoughts and you will feel and be happier.

Point Three Your emotions are the window to your body and soul. I want you to take stock of your emotions everyday. How do you feel today? Your emotions are your antennae to your inner alignment. Your emotions will tell you if your thoughts are properly aligned with your feelings. If your thoughts are taking you in the right direction that's best suited for you, then your emotions will feel positive. Conversely, if your thoughts are moving in a direction that is not right for you, then your emotional antennae will let you know by the way that you feel. Listen to your heart.

Point Four Be confident with the new you. You need not act out life based on what someone else tells you to do, or what you think you should do, or what some institution commands is right for you. The 'shoulds' and the 'oughts' are fantasy. Listening to the dictates of others only displaces your alignment with your thought and feelings. There is only one way to know what is best for you and how to act on your behalf: Look within and feel your inner thoughts and emotions. Feel your soul, your inner core. Listen to the deepest you. Then you will know what is right for you, how to think and when to act.

Let me share a story of my own with you. Not too long ago, I was scheduled to take a trip abroad. I thought that I had to go. It was all planned. Other people were counting on me to show up. And even my own head said 'you've go to go there'. But in a very quiet moment of stillness, I knew in my gut that it did not feel right. I even said to a colleague, 'I know that I should take this trip, but in my belly I feel it will be wrong.'

So my thoughts and feelings were not aligned. I was out of sync with myself. Worse yet, I ignored my feeling of not wanting to go. As it turned out, this would prove to be the trip from a nightmare. On every level, from the terrible airplane ride to horrific weather conditions to scheduling mishaps, everything went wrong, and not just for the one day but for all four days.

Point Five You attract in life the very same vibrations that you personally vibrate. Give out good energy and you will attract good energy. If you vibrate energies of sadness, anger, fear, disappointment, frustration, blame, resentment and the like, then you will attract these same negative energies toward you. Negative energy can manifest in all shapes, sizes and forms, and I have discovered in practice that when people vibrate negative energy, they will be far more likely to make poor food choices. And conversely, when you are feeling happy and thinking positive, you will be more susceptible to making the right healthy food choices. Likewise, when you eat healthy foods, you are likely to feel and think in a more positive and clear way. Happy thoughts attract good food choices and vice versa – the perfect cycle of Ultimate Health.

Point Six Every day (and actually every moment of life) is a new day and a new moment for you to re-create yourself. In other words, just because you had ratty thoughts yesterday doesn't mean that you need them today. Or if your thoughts were out of sync with your feelings earlier today, then in the evening you can still choose to get back into harmony. For instance, you have a fight with your partner before you both leave for work. You know that you still feel the intense love for each other. When you both return home, you decide to kiss and make-up. You have made a conscious choice here to change the energy between the two of you via the thought and actions of resolution. You can use this application in any aspect of your life. You can literally switch on positive or switch off negative thoughts if you make a conscious decision to do so.

Point Seven The bottom line here is that you can change your life. You can make choices and eliminate resistance. You get to decide: good food, positive lifestyle, wellness, great body, slim figure, unconditional love, joy, fulfillment, happiness . . . ultimate health. It's all in your hands.

Wishing you Love & Light,

Gillian

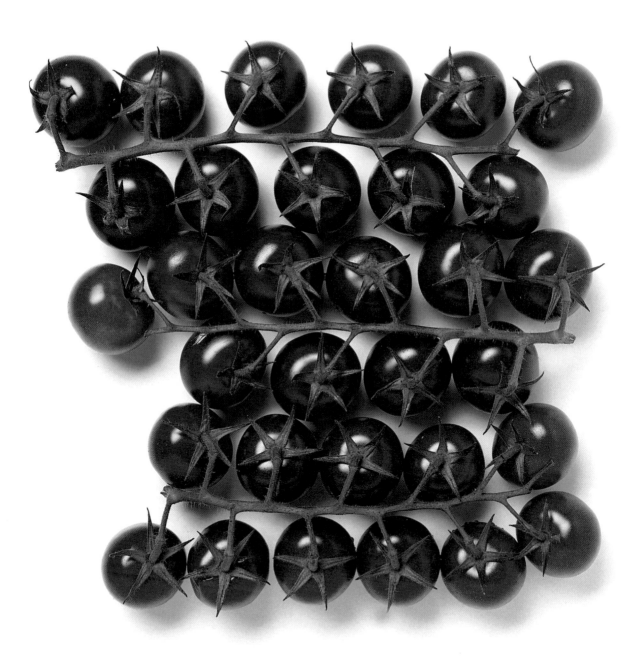

Index

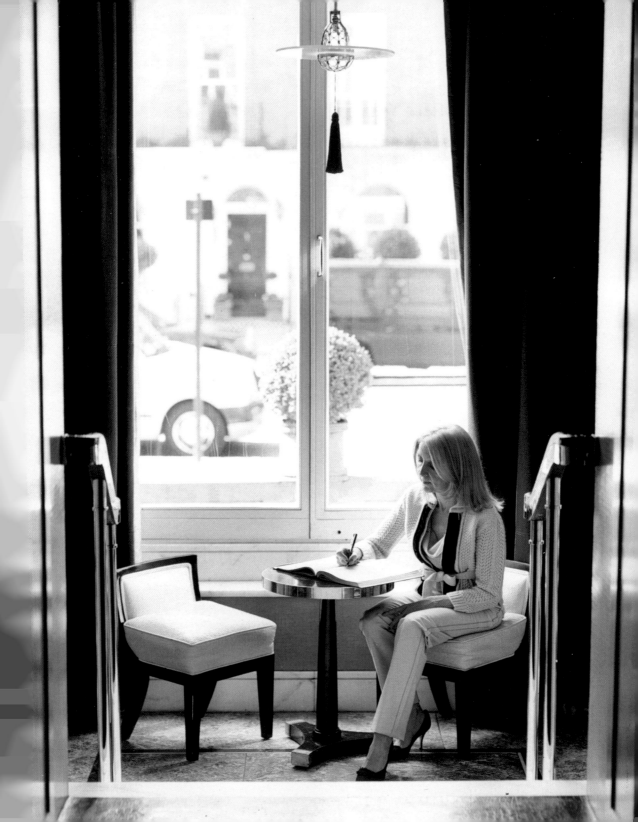

Dear Dad: This book is dedicated to you Dad. Miss you so much. But I feel you close and know you are watching over. Your signs have reaffirmed for me that there is more to life than what we can see, feel, think, touch and smell.

Squeezes, hugs, kisses, cuddles and love to my two wee lassies. You are so loved and cherished. And to my immense, outstanding foundation and inspiration, Howard: You are a gifted catalyst for transformation of the planet on so many levels. Your motivation, huge support, passion, words, and contributions are life-altering and deeply appreciated.

I wish to thank every person who has opened one of my books, flicked on the switch to watch the You Are What You Eat television series or written me a letter of blessing. It is each and every one of you who are making it possible to get my message out to the world.

Enormous gratitude, thanks and love to my editor Kate Adams. You are an exceptional person whose heart and soul is also in this book. Your commitment is inspiring. And to everyone at Smith & Gilmour. Thank you for your tremendous hard work – your design is superb and your creativity unmatched. And thank you to all at Penguin, particularly Tom Weldon, Louise Moore and Sarah Rollason.

Deep appreciation to Helen T. Big hugs to your kids and hubby too. We know our grams inside out now.

Nicola, you are so special and along with Julia, Jo, Dawn, Johnny, Gina, Helen, you are a tremendous team. You all hold a warm place in my heart. THANK YOU for everything. And dearest Luigi: You are an absolute gem.

To my wonderful Max Clifford, much love. Your guidance and kindness is unsurpassed. And to the fantastic Lucy, Louise, Jessica and all at MCA. You are doing wonders.

Big thanks to Theresa for your in-depth research. And to Josie for your excellent support.

Justine. You are a fabulous creative mind.

Thanks to Zdrafka and Izabela for keeping it all together and trying out recipe after recipe. Adzuki Bean Bake. It rocks!!

Oscar, you are still getting me from A to B on time, even when I am not. And dispensing words of wisdom in the process.

To my rocks, Doug and Eloise, a big hug. Gratitude to George, Paul, David, Placy, Leonora and the gang.

To my pillars of strength at McKeith Research Ltd: Non-edible treats take on a whole new meaning with you Alan. You are an incredible individual. Alan, Rob, Indranie and Jon: You are spearheading a movement of enormous change. You are all always there for me, towers of strength. Words don't do justice to how much I am grateful for all that you do.

Chaim Solomon: You get me through and keep me on my spiritual path. You are remarkable.

Much love to Mum. Your encouragement keeps me going strong.

www.drgillianmckeith.com

The Dr Gillian McKeith website is designed to be the ultimate source for active support, help and information. It brings the whole Dr Gillian philosophy to life.

Come on over to the website and discover slimming support, diet help, nutritional information, allergy testing, resource guides, the McKeith Research Centre, free e-newsletters, Live Chat, the Dr Gillian Website Club, and a one-stop shop.

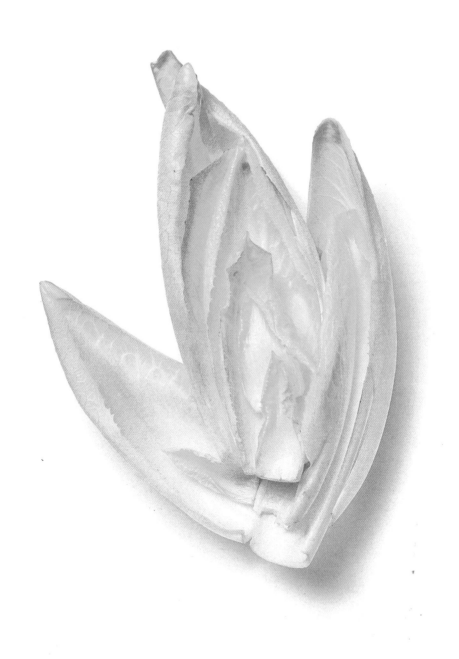